I0416098

Seducing the Burks

Five Erotic Tales

By

Cardyn Brooks

This book is a work of fiction. Places, events, and situations in this story are purely fictional. Any resemblance to actual persons, living or dead, is coincidental.

© 2003 by Cardyn Brooks. All rights reserved.

No part of this book may be reproduced, stored in a retrieval system, or transmitted by any means, electronic, mechanical, photocopying, recording, or otherwise, without written permission from the author.

ISBN: 1-4107-0954-X (e-book)
ISBN: 1-4107-0955-8 (Paperback)

Library of Congress Control Number: 2002096919

This book is printed on acid free paper.

Printed in the United States of America
Bloomington, IN

1stBooks - rev. 06/19/03

Dedication

Thank you to my Individual Encouragement of the Arts team.

Table of Contents

Author's Note

This is a work of fiction. Names, characters, places, and incidents are either the product of the author's imagination or are used fictitiously. Any resemblance to actual persons, living or dead, business establishments, events or locales is entirely coincidental.

Erotic fiction creates a fantasy world where the consequences of high risk behavior are not actually life-threatening. In real life, heed the warnings and recommendations of legitimate physicians and health experts.

FIRST CHOICE

Friday afternoon

Jessamine Winterberry. Who finally satisfied Derrick Bailif two weekends ago? Ask him.

Each of the three times it repeated, the message remained the same. I saved it. Nothing threatening came up in my e-link when I checked. A quick call to my home voice mail yielded incoherent messages of demand from my dad and two of my three older sisters—as if I could influence Mom's actions any more than they could. At least the anonymous informant called only the direct line to my dinky set designer's office in the county playhouse rather than breaching my private domain.

The room spun. My stomach rolled. Innocent until proven guilty, I reminded myself. Don't call his office. Wait until we see each other tonight.

* * *

Paolo's on the South River was crowded, but the hostess still seated us at our favorite table where we'd celebrated his promotions and my favorable notices.

Lush colors, decadent fabrics, glittering place settings, and the view of the river created the perfect environment for enjoying five-star Eastern Shore cuisine.

Our entrées arrived before I found the nerve to ask.

* * *

"Derrick, did you take a lover two weekends ago?"

His ridiculously long dark lashes brushed his cheeks when his eyelids fluttered—his only visible sign of surprise.

"Yes, Jessamine, I slept with a colleague during the management retreat weekend. We were discreet."

As if discretion mitigated the pain of betrayal.

His speculative gaze and refusal to explain angered me. Before the start of our year-long dating relationship I'd told Derrick that my abstinence from sexual intercourse wasn't a ploy or a gimmick, but was my only guarantee against pregnancy, disease, and confusing sex with trust.

He'd agreed. He respected me. Insisted on dating me. Six months later he declared us a monogamous couple: He stopped dating other women. I'd dated him exclusively from the beginning.

So many questions hovered behind my closed lips while this beautiful man had the nerve to smile into my eyes.

"Jessamine." Derrick placed his hand over mine in the center of the table. "Your hands are wonderful, but no substitute for the real thing." He laced our fingers. Tightened his grip when I tugged.

My questions could wait. Time to escape. Call a taxi. Make it easy for this Great Catch to be with the owner of the disembodied sultry voice on my answering machine. Did the servers and other diners sense my humiliation? Were they slyly watching as Derrick shifted responsibility for his betrayal?

"Sexually, I need more than you've offered so far. Your inexperience keeps you from knowing what you're missing. Marry me, Jessie. As your husband I'd never stray."

No remorse. No apologies. A marriage proposal minus the ring. Somehow a ceremony and a piece of paper would make him faithful until something else caused him to dishonor his word.

Smiling, I leaned toward him.

"I know what it is to want a solid erection connected to a male body thrusting inside me instead of fantasies, fingers, and inanimate substitutes." My free hand shoved my plate of food across the table. His wine flute wobbled then tipped into his lap. Now he tried to release me but I refused.

"You vindictive Puritan tease," he whispered.

We battled silently. Both of us attempting to keep our drama private.

My plate teetered at the edge until it plopped into his lap. Crab, lobster, decorative roughage, and olive oil joined the wine. Derrick jerked backward when I released his hand.

"Stay put," he hissed as I gathered my purse.

I scooted out of my seat and stood.

"I haven't dated a man I'd trust with my heart, much less my body. Goodbye, Derrick." My stomach lurched.

I forced myself to glide between the tables. I heard our server fussing over the mishap. In the foyer the hostess signaled the concierge to summon a taxi at my request, then retrieved my over-size silk scarf from the cloak room. By the time Derrick appeared at the entrance I had just locked the taxi's backdoor.

* * *

At the side door to the playhouse I gave the driver a big tip for detouring through the liquor store drive-through.

Inside my office I placed my liters of mixed berry juice and black currant vodka on the desk, then searched for a cup.

Someone knocked.

I wondered if coming here to avoid another confrontation with Derrick might have put me in danger.

"Hello?" The knob jiggled. "Jessamine?"

I recognized Alonzo Burk's voice.

"I'm fine, Alonzo. Just doing some paperwork. Goodnight." As the building maintenance coordinator he knew that my creative workspace was a studio behind the stage.

His silence concerned me, especially when the knob slowly turned back and forth.

Almost a minute later, he asked, "Do you trust me, Jessamine?"

"Yes, of course, Alonzo."

We had met three years earlier at the city soup kitchen where we both volunteered on Tuesday afternoons. Months later I'd encouraged him to bid for the opportunity for his fourth-generation company, Burk Family Plumbing and Building Maintenance, to serve the playhouse.

"Then show yourself. Unlock this door."

I dabbed at my eyes and very quietly blew my nose into my crumpled handkerchief. Deep breathing calmed me a little as I crossed the office.

"Hi." My smile felt painfully wide.

Alonzo executed a swift one-eyed inspection of me and the room.

"Why are you crying and planning to get drunk?"

For his every step forward I backtracked two until my hips hit the edge of my desk nearly toppling my beverages.

Even with the patch over his left eye, and the patchwork of scars covering that side of his face and neck, I didn't fear him. During the years of our acquaintance he'd never said anything or acted in a way that frightened me.

"What's happened, Jessamine?"

That single perfect brown eye just stared at me. The heat from his strong body drew me. We leaned toward each other at the same instant.

"Personal drama." I burrowed into his tight embrace. "A few hours of self-pity and liquor are all I need." The stroke of his hand over my disheveled hair soothed me. "Why are you here?"

"Another burst pipe." His breath caressed my ear.

I'd heard that a group of anonymous benefactors had pledged money for new pipes to be fitted, but the funds wouldn't be available for several weeks.

"I was doing a final walk-through when I saw the light under your door."

Surrounded by the tenor of his voice and the feel of his body, his presence muted the evening's earlier discord.

* * *

For the first time since winning the community playhouse contract, Alonzo thanked fate for the deteriorated condition of the building's plumbing. He hadn't foreseen that a nine-one-one page from the custodian would result in the realization of three years of fantasies about getting close to Jessamine Winterberry.

While her voluptuous body settled into his embrace Alonzo reminded himself to proceed with caution. Finding a weepy woman locked in a room with a liter of liquor suggested devastating news—probably a lovers' quarrel.

Just when he'd decided to coax the details from Jessamine, her warm plump lips pressed a kiss to the fabric over his breastbone. His nerves jumped, reminding him that he hadn't held a woman in more than three years. He'd paid the sex worker even though her poorly hidden revulsion had rendered him temporarily impotent. That was the last time he'd worked up the nerve to pursue a woman with his sexual interests.

Jessamine's tight embrace and roaming lips tempted Alonzo to accept what she offered without asking any questions. He resisted.

"Jessamine?" He pried her arms from his waist. "What happened tonight?" Spinning their positions, Alonzo propped his hips against her desk before settling her body between his hard thighs. His muscular arms bound their torsos together. Her tears soaked his shirt collar. "Quarrel with your lover?"

* * *

Alonzo's question released all the pain I wanted to ignore. He asked again and I started sobbing, wetting his shirt front. Raised flesh rubbed my cheek beneath the damp cotton twill fabric.

Before we'd ever met, I'd heard his name during news broadcasts when he had been found alive after being buried under tons of glass and metal for two days.

9

A corporate site under construction had collapsed because of sub-standard materials. Eight people were killed.

Alonzo's embrace pinned my arms to my sides. He kept whispering in my ear; prompting me to share my secrets with him.

I stretched up to kiss him, just to silence him.

* * *

She was rebounding. Alonzo felt it in the desperation of her kiss. He should resist. Take her home. But he hadn't kissed a woman with sensual intent in more than three years. He loosened his hold to bring his hands to her cheeks, to frame her face.

The taste of her obliterated coherent thought beyond taking his fill. He ravaged her mouth. Nibbled her gloriously full lips until she moaned. He trapped her hands at the small of her back when she attempted to embrace him.

"Let me touch you," she said between kisses.

Alonzo responded by pulling her astride one of his heavily muscled thighs. The sudden, intense pleasure startled her into gasping. His tongue filled her open mouth while the strength of his hands pressed her mons into his thigh.

He placed her hands on his shoulders, then ended the kiss. Jessamine's dazed eyes returned his harsh stare. "If you move your hands, I'll stop. Understand?" He doubted any event short of Armageddon or her withdrawal could stop him.

Alonzo knew Jessamine was using him. What better retaliation against her pretty-boy professional than to have a quickie with the ugliest man she knows? Lust and doubt battled for primacy. Should he indulge her knowing that afterward she might despise him and herself?

He would create a way to sample her body without losing their friendship.

* * *

His fierce expression scared me, but my desire was greater than my fear. Suddenly this man who had always treated me like a beloved little sister was overwhelming me with his sexual pull. Being desired so much intensified my excitement.

11

My fingers clutched his shoulders. I kissed him to show my acceptance of his terms and everything he offered—especially the chance to forget the outside world for a short time. Maybe later he'd accept my touch.

His large sculptured hands grabbed my hips and dragged me higher into the notch of his thighs and groin. My short skirt rose revealing plain black garters and lacy panties. I twisted in his embrace, but couldn't escape his tongue thrusting into my mouth or his fingers kneading my buttocks, rocking my clitoris against sturdy denim and rubbing my tender breasts against his solid pectorals. Every muscle between my legs clenched around unbearable emptiness. Slick moisture lay wasted on my inner thighs. I turned my head gasping for breath. Alonzo tilted me backward, took my right breast into his mouth—dress, bra, and all. I screamed. My hold on his shirt threatened to rip its seams.

Alonzo shoved his thigh higher and clutched my buttocks tighter, grinding my sex against his leg. I fainted.

* * *

Seconds before Jessamine slumped in his arms, Alonzo considered the possibility of using this sexual encounter as an initial step toward a deeper relationship. He hoped their solid years-long friendship would balance the fact that she was rebounding. He needed details of what he guessed was her sudden break-up with the poster boy for corporate achievement. He and Derrick had never moved beyond the cordiality of strangers the few times they'd met at the soup kitchen, playhouse fundraisers, and Jessamine's parties.

Juggling Jessamine into a one-armed hug, Alonzo pulled a handkerchief from his back pocket. He was glad she remained unconscious while he sopped the moisture glistening on her pubes and inner thighs. For a brief moment the temptation to ease one finger into the source of her musky fragrance lured him until a glimpse at her vulnerable body returned him to sanity. Emotional overload probably contributed to her fainting as much as his sexual prowess, but he took satisfaction from her shattered response anyway. The large wet spot on his jeans proved that he'd excited her.

Lifting her hips, Alonzo tugged the scrap of lace free of her swollen labia, then straightened her silk-lined skirt and pulled until the hem draped a few inches above her knees. He shifted her to his other thigh to save her skirt from the wet spot. He rocked her in his embrace while he waited for her unfathomable eyes to open.

* * *

My first conscious thought was that Derrick was right: I am a Puritan tease. The warmth and hardness of Alonzo's erection nudged my hip through our layers of clothes.

I forced my eyes open expecting to see anger in his face instead of the look of intense concentration with which he regarded me. That's when I realized he'd cleaned my body and straightened my clothes in addition to pleasuring me into oblivion.

Why wasn't he berating me?

"Where, Jessamine?"

Grabbing my hands when I reached toward his face, he twisted his scarred side away from me. He was still unwilling for me to see or touch his tightly stretched and stitched flesh. I decided to reciprocate pleasure for pleasure; to take him to my home and seduce him.

"Home."

* * *

Alonzo double-parked while I ran into the pharmacy for condoms, lubricant, and Epsom salts. He thought I needed pain reliever and a cold pack for my headache and swollen eyes.

* * *

Alonzo felt equal parts joy and fear when Jessamine led him into her home, then disappeared down the central hall. His eyes scanned the inviting atmosphere.

Seeing the interior without the press of gyrating bodies or seated dinner guests allowed him to appreciate the cool colors and clean lines of her three-bedroom bungalow. Half-burned candles of various sizes and shapes accented every flat surface. Traces of their fragrance lingered in the air. Many windows combined with the open floor plan fostered a sense of space.

Jessamine reappeared with her face freshly scrubbed. From his seat in one of her over-stuffed lounge chairs he watched her mute the ringer on the phone before mixing their drinks. She appeared much calmer. Maybe he'd take a few sips, then leave. He could call her over the weekend: Invite himself over or invite her out as a friendly overture of concern; solidify this encounter as a foundation for something deeper with Jessamine. Earlier his scars hadn't repelled her, but she had been concentrating on other things. He couldn't predict how she'd respond under normal circumstances. He was too weary to speculate. Too aroused to squash the budding hope their office encounter had planted in his heart. He needed to be alone with his fist and an icy shower before he exploded.

* * *

Getting him tipsy seemed the best way to make him stay, but I didn't know how much alcohol would affect such a muscular man. I'd made his drink mostly vodka with a little juice. Mine was all juice.

"I should go. Give you some quiet time."

Alonzo drained his glass. I hoped he hadn't eaten much during the day.

"Please stay. An evening of self-pity no longer appeals to me."

He allowed me to refresh his drink. His body appeared less rigidly held than when he'd first taken a seat. In the past three years I had never seen Alonzo do more than nurse one mixed drink throughout an entire social event. No matter how he appeared, he was probably too affected by alcohol consumption to drive home safely. The second drink should convince him to spend the night.

"Thank you for tonight, Alonzo. I would have been hung-over and embarrassed if someone had found me at the playhouse tomorrow morning."

"Glad to help." His beautiful eye stared at me. "But would you have trusted your body to any man who'd shown up at the playhouse, or do you trust me specifically?"

* * *

A minute too late Alonzo remembered why he had never been a drinker, especially on an empty stomach— empty calories and loose lips.

One of Jessamine's hands fluttered near her face. She coughed. She sipped her drink. Finally she said, "I trust you specifically. I've never climaxed that quickly or strongly before being in your arms tonight." She rubbed the ends of her hair. "Would you have comforted any woman that way, or did my identity matter?"

Jessamine watched him roll his glass between his palms. His gaze drifted from her face to linger at her breasts where his mouth had put a faint water mark. He studied her legs demurely crossed at the ankles, then finished his drink. He decided to tell the truth.

"I want you, Jessamine. I've wanted you for some time, but I'm willing to wait until you've dealt with whatever happened with Derrick tonight. My goal is to be more than some consolation lover."

Alonzo damned himself as a fool for making demands when he should be grateful for whatever

Jessamine was willing to give. His imagination produced images of her running from the sight of his scarred body. He shook his head, focused on the reality of the lush beauty seated within reach. Silently he dared her to accept him and his new terms.

* * *

The future seemed too complicated, but I knew that giving him pleasure was my only immediate concern. I set aside each of our glasses before kneeling between his spread thighs. My hands hovered over his legs. He didn't react when I clasped his thighs. He didn't object when my hands roamed over the finely developed musculature of his legs. My eyes followed the path of my hands, but the weight of his stare pressed against the crown of my bent head. I looked up to face his terrible beauty.

"Derrick is my past. You are my present, Alonzo. You're no consolation lover, but an unexpected gift." I leaned forward to press my lips against the scarred side of his face. His erection nudged my pelvis. I performed a slow, hard grind, which forced a throaty moan from him. "Stay the night with me, Alonzo."

I interpreted his open-mouthed kiss over my lips, and groping hands on my buttocks as a yes.

* * *

A chance to have sex for the first time in three years—with the woman of his choice. Alonzo's mind short-circuited, but his body shifted into automatic pilot. The two drinks had only taken the edge off his painful readiness. He put his shoulder to Jessamine's midriff and hoisted her into a firefighter's carry. Her hands clutched his back while Alonzo stalked through her house until he found her bedroom where a lamp glowed softly on her vanity table. He approached the queen-size bed.

She bounced once after he tossed her onto the mattress. Jessamine scrambled to her knees before he could cover her with his aroused body.

"Second thoughts?" he asked after sucking in some deep breaths. He watched her reach toward the condoms on the nightstand. In his haste he would have had her legs spread and sex full before protection would have occurred to him.

Jessamine crept toward him. Alonzo fisted his hands behind his back barely controlling his need to strip her and possess her without any preliminaries. He held his breath while Jessamine loosened his belt and unfastened his fly. Warm, smooth hands pushed his briefs and jeans down to his ankles. Fear of rejection tempted him to shove her away, run outside, jump into his truck, and return to the safety of his home. He felt her tentatively cup his tightly drawn sac in one hand. The other palmed his rigid sex. A minute later latex gloved his erection before she swallowed him.

* * *

I nearly gagged when he thrust against the back of my throat. It didn't take us long to coordinate a mutually pleasurable rhythm. He was resisting his orgasm. His grunts rose in pitch, volume, and frequency as I licked and sucked his engorged penis while my hands squeezed his testicles. He came hard and fast, shouting my name and jerking free of my mouth and hands. He

21

collapsed with his chest on the bed, his knees on the floor. I stroked the side of his face while he gasped for breath. Wads of comforter twisted in his clenched fists.

He helped me drag him onto the bed when I grabbed his shirt collar and pulled. I decided we should be naked.

* * *

Alonzo opened his eyes to see her supple breasts tenuously confined in a lacy black confection masquerading as a brassiere. The longer he stared, the faster her breasts moved. Her nipples poked the decadent lace.

He forced his gaze up to her eyes.

"I've indulged myself with pretty lingerie since my first job in high school," she said.

Alonzo thought about her usual attire of baggy trousers and tailored shirts.

"You always wear these types of undergarments?"

"Yes."

He allowed her to shift toward his feet to remove his boots, jeans, briefs, and used latex because her position gave him a perfect view of her luscious backside covered in lace and framed by garters. He was glad she wore her panties over her garter belt.

The light touch of her lips on the patchwork of lines and gouges across his legs shifted his focus. Her hands caressed the soles of his feet, massaging the arches until he gave an involuntary chuckle.

Intending retribution, Alonzo hauled her up to face him. She dropped against his body with a thud. The sight of her watery eyes enraged him.

"Pity?"

Jessamine shook her head. "Joy that you survived," she whispered.

Alonzo wondered if her face radiated truth because she spoke it, or because he wanted it. The musk of her arousal filled his nostrils. Why couldn't he just take her body without understanding her motives?

He watched her graceful fingers slip his buttons free one by one until she laid his chest bare. She smiled into his eye despite the tears slowly rolling down her cheeks.

"You're the strongest person I know."

* * *

Could I give him enough pleasure to cancel the pain his scars testified that he had endured? I had to try.

I reached between my breasts to unfasten my bra, but Alonzo stopped me.

"Leave it."

He arranged himself with his limbs spread wide after he shrugged out of his shirt. His posture indicated surrender while his eyes projected victory. His hands fisted as I reached for his eye patch slowly, giving him every opportunity to stop me.

* * *

Alonzo thought letting Jessamine see his body unclothed would end all his chances of being her lover. The feel of her moist lips against the lid sown over his empty eye socket jolted his senses. His hope grew.

Jessamine's tender lips and gentle hands caressed the whole surface of his skin, lingering over waxy smooth areas, keloidal masses, and puckered gaps. Her tears bathed him when she pressed her face against his flesh to inhale his existence.

Jessamine's physical affection was the first he had received from a non-family member in more than three years. Tenderness grew from each point of contact between them. Alonzo would do anything to claim all of Jessamine for himself.

* * *

His long stretch of passivity lulled me into a languid mood. Only his guttural moans told me how he felt. I began thinking of his body as my personal domain.

He pounced. My delicate panties were ripped from my crotch, my legs spread as widely as possible, and my arms pinned to the mattress before I recognized my vulnerability to his coiled energy.

"Last chance for regrets, Jessamine. Do you choose to be my lover?"

His hard penis jabbed the base of my clit sending tremors of anticipation through me.

"Yes."

Alonzo's tongue deeply penetrated my mouth.

* * *

He would brand her so deeply with himself that any future regrets would be insignificant and fleeting. Their shared pleasure would bind her to him.

He reached for another condom and sheathed his erection without breaking their kiss. One finger eased inside her tight, wet channel, which clamped around his digit like strong suction. His penis twitched in anticipation of being milked dry.

His other hand trapped both of her wrists over her head.

"Raise your knees to your chest."

The novelty of his harsh command shocked her into compliance. The compression of her vagina shifted the feel of his invading finger from pleasure to pain.

Alonzo withdrew his finger because the sight of her pouty vulva and curvy buttocks enticed him to taste.

"Grab these." He wrapped her fingers around the spindles of her headboard. "Don't release them."

His hands slid down her arms, shoulders, breasts, and waist until he placed them around her thighs to keep her body folded and her sex exposed. She

26

climaxed as soon as his tongue penetrated her nether lips and his nose brushed the underside of her clit. Her keening cry spiraled to an earsplitting pitch, then faded into panting breaths.

Alonzo braced her tucked legs with one forearm while he worked one thick finger into her quivering vagina, preparing her to accept his stiff penis within the next half minute.

She whimpered in discomfort when he attempted to introduce a second finger alongside the first.

"Not including me, Jessamine, how many lovers have you taken?" He idly peered at her clenched anus before he glanced at her face.

"None." Receding waves of orgasm tightened the walls around his finger. "I'm virgin."

* * *

Had wishful thinking distorted his hearing? The clutch of her body around his single penetrating digit supported the likelihood of her claim. He'd never been anyone's sexual initiator. Knowing he could take her blotted just about every other thought from his mind. Beneath him her body trembled with strain. Her sex

27

wept for the promise of being filled with his erection. Alonzo struggled not to ram her untried body. His every instinct screamed at him to possess her body to guarantee an irrevocable claim. The strong draw of her fragrance threatened to fog his brain.

"Alonzo, you're hurting me."

Her breathy whisper made him aware of how he had dropped all of his weight against her folded body while his finger worked its way deeper between the walls of her tender tissue.

"Release her," the reasonable portion of his mind chanted.

* * *

A scream was gathering momentum in my throat when Alonzo finally withdrew his finger and lifted himself from my body. I inhaled deeply for the first time since he had ordered me to raise my knees.

Although he handled me gently while he unfolded my legs and loosened my fingers from the headboard, his hard facial expression concerned me until he leaned forward to press chaste kisses against the corners of my mouth.

Some men avoid sexual involvement with virgins because of the potential for emotional entanglement. Alonzo's sudden tenderness made me think my virginity had cooled his enthusiasm even though his erection felt solid and hot against my thigh when he reclined and held me alongside him. Tension quivered along the surface of his skin.

Now I regretted telling him, but if he had thrust his penis into my compressed vagina with the same force he used with his fingers, he would have hurt me—virgin or not.

Gradually Alonzo's muscles relaxed. His breathing quieted.

* * *

Alonzo decided that a woman like Jessamine who unconditionally offered him affection and her virginity only hours after some type of major emotional upset deserved his consideration no matter how much his body rejected the idea. Before he accepted such irrevocable gifts from Jessamine, he needed details.

29

"Tell me what happened before I found you barricaded inside your office."

* * *

I told him everything beginning with the mystery woman's message and ending with my running from Derrick at the restaurant.

Sunlight peaked around the edges of my Roman shades. I eased from Alonzo's embrace, got out of bed, and switched off the lamp. Being naked made me self-conscious. I shrugged into Alonzo's shirt, fragrant with his unique scent. A faint impression of my lips rendered in dark chocolate #3 showed on the front placket. Thoughts of all the places on his body Alonzo had allowed me to kiss made me smile.

Weak light filtered into the room once I raised the shades. Privacy glass prevented anyone outside from seeing us.

On my way back to bed Alonzo said, "Thank you for trusting me with your secrets." He held his arms out to me as he yawned. "Let's nap."

We slept past noon.

* * *

Derrick Bailif pressed the doorbell for the third time, faintly hearing it chime inside Jessamine's small house.

After last night's embarrassing scene at the restaurant Derrick had been too enraged to see or speak to Jessamine. He'd driven around listening to music and berating himself for not honoring Lydia's terms. She had seen Jessamine with Derrick at various company social events during the past year. Before Lydia had agreed to have sex with him during the retreat weekend, she had made him swear to tell Jessamine about the affair. He'd assumed that Jessamine's unlisted unpublished home phone number and inconsistent hours at the playhouse would prevent Lydia from contacting Jessamine.

He had underestimated Lydia's resourcefulness. There were reasons why she was one of the company's top five revenue producers.

He pressed the bell again.

His attention focused on the year-old luxury extended cab pickup parked in Jessamine's driveway. He didn't recognize it as belonging to her parents, her sisters, or any of her closest friends, but anyone could be visiting at almost one o' clock on a Saturday afternoon.

The door opened. Jessamine peered at him through the locked storm door. Derrick scanned her appearance from tousled hair and cleanly scrubbed face to unfamiliar, wrinkled man's shirt, leggings, and bare feet. His gaze lingered on her painted toes before returning to her direct gaze.

"Invite me inside."

"Speak your mind, then go, Derrick."

"No."

She stepped backward in order to close the inner steel door.

"Fine." Derrick stepped closer to the transparent barrier. "You should have heard about the retreat weekend from me. I apologize for yielding to temptation. Let's start fresh. Today. This minute."

* * *

I realized we had been mismatched from the start. Neither one of us was what the other one desired. I'd used him to silence my family's and other people's questions about my romantic future. Derrick's combination of desirable attributes made him a good man, but the wrong man for me.

I wanted him to leave before Alonzo came searching for me.

"Your coworker's appeal to you was stronger than your commitment to our relationship. Last night forced both of us out of denial. Let's part as friends. Okay?"

Derrick scowled fiercely at me. His eyes raked me from head to toe more than once.

"Who's with you, Jess?"

I considered shutting the door.

"A friend."

"Male or female?"

It was none of his business, but some mean-spirited aspect of my personality wanted him to know.

"Male."

"Is this retribution? Who is he, Jess?"

I shouldn't have answered the door.

"Goodbye, Derrick."

* * *

Alonzo found Jessamine sitting huddled against the front door. She raised her head when he knelt before her. He doubted she could see him clearly through her swollen red eyes.

"He stood on the porch for about ten minutes after you closed the door."

Jessamine frowned. "When did you wake?"

Alonzo leaned forward gathering her into his arms. "As soon as the bell rang."

She burrowed as close to him as possible, pressing her cheek against his bare shoulder.

"All cried out?" Alonzo asked. His breath skimmed the top of her head. His powerful arms crisscrossed her back.

Jessamine sniffled. "I hope." Alonzo strained to hear her voice. "If you hadn't been here, I would have let him in."

He loosened his embrace and raised her chin with the edge of his hand. Alonzo smiled into her bleary eyes.

"Then my being here was a good thing." His thumb caressed her jawline. "The first time is always most difficult when saying goodbye to the safety of what's familiar."

Jessamine jabbed one finger into his chest. "Derrick's got some nerve thinking he can just appear," she snapped her fingers, "and act as if nothing happened." She huffed and crossed her arms beneath her breasts. "That man is bold."

"From where I sit, knowing you merits any amount of boldness. I can't fault Derrick for trying, Jessamine."

Her sudden smile warmed him.

"What a charming opinion, Alonzo. Thank you."

She pressed a kiss to his sown eyelid. He marveled at her ability to view his face and body without disgust. Her lips drifted across his features while her hands stroked whatever naked flesh she could reach.

"My past is reconciled, Alonzo." Her tongue rimmed the shell of his ear. "You're still my first choice."

Their limbs tangled and bumped until Jessamine sat astride his kneeling body, embracing him loosely, and staring into his battered face.

"I want you," she whispered as she performed a slow grind over his obvious erection. "You want me too."

Alonzo's agonized groan echoed around them. He thought he might ejaculate in his jeans for the first time in his life.

* * *

He panted as if he had run a four-minute mile. His resistance was weakening. These hours with Alonzo had given me a deeper appreciation for how much effort men have to expend to get sexed.

The way he stared at the deep cleavage his shirt created on my chest inspired me to bare my breasts and pull his head down until his lips nuzzled then suckled. His fingers gripped my buttocks, jamming my sex against the hard protrusion confined behind his fly. Alonzo stopped me when I tried to strip off my leggings.

* * *

Despite his rapidly cresting orgasm and Jessamine's determined struggles to undress them both, Alonzo managed to think beyond the moment. He decided to use sex to lure Jessamine into a relationship. He would court her mind; tantalize her body until she offered him her virginity as a gesture of commitment rather than as an act of defiance. Because regardless of Jessamine's sincere words, Alonzo knew her current determination to take him as her first lover was as much a response to Derrick's actions as it was a manifestation of some attraction to Alonzo. She was rebounding—whether or not she recognized it. In the meantime, Alonzo would avoid coitus to hedge against possible regrets, and as a way to preserve her virginity even if only by a technicality.

Guiding her legs around his waist, Alonzo stood. Without removing his mouth from her breasts he slowly carried her to her bedroom.

* * *

For hours Alonzo drove me into successive orgasms finally leaving me too sated to move. Almost too relaxed to keep my eyes open to study how he pleasured himself. My sex throbbed swollen and raw between my legs even though we had used lubricant. The surface of my skin tingled with hypersensitivity. Alonzo's mouth, fingers, and toes had worked me over, making even the thought of touching myself painful. I'd remain barely virgin for one more day.

"On your side." His harsh words startled me, but his hands flipped me before I could move.

Exhaustion kept me from being alarmed when he raised my top leg. Like caulking a seam, his latex covered pulsing sex filled the length of my vulva without entering me. Pubic hair tickled my buttocks before he pressed my legs together wedging his penis tightly between my sex and thighs. He braced one arm across the tops of my thighs to trap my hips while he sawed back and forth, forcing my mound against his forearm. I moaned.

"Squeeze your glutes, Jessamine." His tight grip would leave bruises. "Press your legs together as hard as you can," Alonzo said in a harsh whisper I had grown accustomed to hearing during the last hour.

The speed and friction of his thrusts burned everywhere he touched. Seconds later his penis jerked between my clenched muscles. His hands slipped over my breasts. Agonizing sensation jolted the connection from my breasts to my clit. Alonzo kept one hand at my breasts. The other drifted down to torment the aroused skin around my aching bud.

Exhaustion combined with the pressure of his body and sexual overload drained my consciousness as I climaxed.

* * *

I awoke to find myself submerged in a tub full of lukewarm water. My eyes wondered into focus on the box of Epsom salts at the foot of the tub. Alonzo's reclining body cradled me. His arms folded beneath my breasts kept my head above water. He had hooked my legs atop his, keeping me open to allow the water to soothe my inflamed sex.

There was no artificial light to interfere with our view of the sunset through the windows along one side of the tub.

"Awake?"

"Yes."

"Thank you for this experience, Jessamine."

"My pleasure, Alonzo."

His soft chuckle rumbled against my back.

"Will you have dinner with me tomorrow night? *The Harlem Quartet* plays second set at *Jazzy's.*"

My limbs felt leaden and disconnected from my brain. My mind floated free of my body, but I would manage to re-connect all my systems to spend more time with Alonzo. "Yes."

TRUE BEAUTY

"Steph, he's too tasty."

Ashley and Antonia jockeyed for the best view of my neighbor while he used manual clippers to shape his hedges. My sisters had salivated over and speculated about Mordecai Burk during each of their visits for the past fourteen months. Since my move from renter to homeowner, I had offered them an open invitation to brunch on the first Saturday of every month.

My older sister and my younger sister shared a familiar look which always preceded embarrassment for me.

They straightened my drapes then gathered their handbags. "We're leaving," they said in unison. "Walk us out."

They were halfway to my driveway before I decided to follow.

* * *

"Hi, Mordecai," they said in answer to his smile and wave.

Ashley said, "Yard work must make you very thirsty. Stephanie has fresh-squeezed lemonade. Have some when you're finished."

Subtlety had always been an alien concept to my big sister. Unfortunately, sink holes weren't common in this part of the country. Thank Creation my complexion hid my blush.

"In fact," my traitorous baby sister said, "help Stephanie eat the remaining portions of the delicious brunch she cooked for us. You've been working for hours; you must be famished."

Ashley ran interference between Antonia and me with her body.

"No guts, no love, Steph. Be bold," Ashley whispered in my ear while we hugged.

When Ashley released me, Antonia bussed each side of my face. "Don't be mad. He's flattered." I said, "In another life I must have been a meddlesome sibling."

They both laughed as they settled into their vehicles.

I waved until their cars disappeared from my sight.

I wondered what to say to Mordecai.

* * *

An hour later he rang my doorbell.

"Come on, Stephanie, I'm starved."

I relented once he started serenading me in Yoruba.

"Get in here!" I yanked him across the threshold and shut the door before our neighbors got curious.

Mordecai spun me into a friendly squeeze that lifted me from the floor. He carried me into the kitchen where he devoured every mouthful of leftover brunch and washed it down with a half-full pitcher of lemonade.

His deeply set dark brown eyes narrowed on my face. "Your sisters don't know we're good friends."

My body initiated a sensual response to his voice even though anger threaded its pitch.

"Mercy, Mordecai, look at how they behave when they believe we're only cordial neighbors."

I stared at his back while he rinsed dishes and loaded the dishwasher. He scrubbed my counters with fierce jerks of his sinewy arm.

"They don't know what began our relationship?"

A year ago I'd made an appointment with him to explain some tax law to me. I'd been gathering information for my sideline job as a researcher for the reclusive novelist R.J. Bakerman. When Mordecai learned that librarian was my full-time occupation, he had asked that I participate in career day at his niece's nursery school instead of paying him cash for his time and knowledge. He wanted his niece and her schoolmates to see brown-skinned women as everything from astronaut to zoologist.

I watched Mordecai clean until my kitchen was spotless. He would speak once he'd worked out his arguments within his mind. He grabbed my hands and backed toward my loveseat in the sun room. He seated himself before tugging me into his lap.

Using the tone of voice I imagined Mordecai used to reprimand his clients who submitted incomplete tax records, he said, "You haven't told your sisters we walk five miles together every morning?"

Mordecai had volunteered to speedwalk with me when a serial rapist terrorized the community last spring. By the time the prime suspect was in custody, we had established a comfortable routine.

I didn't shift my gaze from his hard stare.

"If Ashley and Antonia knew the depth of our friendship, they would harass you until you proposed marriage, filed a complaint or moved."

Mordecai and I shared season tickets for the state dance theater, and NFL franchise. We had exchanged housekeys and alarm codes for emergencies and deliveries. We frequently escorted each other to work-related social engagements.

He did not return my half-hearted smile.

"Stephanie, you've met many of my clients, my family, and my closest friends without introducing me to anyone other than your coworkers. Your sisters introduced themselves to me." A muscle near the corner of his left eye twitched the way it does whenever Mordecai is annoyed with me. "Are you ashamed of me?"

As if the woman voted *most likely to break a mirror without touching it* could be ashamed of the wise, intelligent, hard-bodied beauty Mordecai Burk personified.

In high school my skin had been riddled with acne. The war between my glands and hormones had raged

45

until my sophomore year of college. By the time my skin cleared I'd mastered the art of friendship without having a clue about the pursuit of romance.

In my mind, Ashley and Antonia were the men magnets. I was the pal, sister, good friend.

I stroked the side of his face until his muscle spasm stopped. "I'm proud to know you. Proud to be your friend. To be seen with you. I just want to hoard our time together, Mordecai. You haven't met my friends because they would hotfoot it over to my sisters quicker than a wink."

Pressing a kiss against his neck did not completely dissolve the sullen cast of his face.

"Invite your sisters to my home for cocktails this Friday evening, Stephanie. Let's introduce them to the idea of our being involved."

He kissed me when I opened my mouth to argue for a postponement. Mordecai's succulent lips brushed mine in several slow feathery passes before the tip of his tongue traced my lower and upper lips and the seam between them. The tantalizing feel of his mouth on mine nearly distracted me from the gentle caress of his strong hands at my waist and breast.

Just beneath the scents of soap and moisturizer the smell of the outdoors clung to his skin and hair. The muscles across his shoulders rippled under my hands as he tipped me onto the cushions and covered my body with his.

Weeks ago I had realized that I loved a man who appeared too beautiful to be attracted to the ugly girl I often believed myself to be regardless of my reflection in the mirror. Sometimes worries that his apparent interest in me was part of some elaborate practical joke undermined my responses to his ardor.

The hard knot of his arousal pressed my stomach through layers of cloth. All my insecurities conspired to suggest that convenient location was my primary appeal. I cancelled my negative thoughts with positive facts: Mordecai desired me. He respected me with his words and actions. I thanked the Universe for everything that knowing him added to my life.

Especially the physical gratification. Mordecai's kisses gradually deepened. He always kissed me as if we had days to spare; as if he were afraid to neglect one millimeter of my lips and mouth. Cool air touched my chest where he had unbuttoned my shirt. One thumb flicked my nipples while his other hand loosened my trousers and slipped inside to hold my buttocks in the firm grasp of his scarred fingers and callous palm, legacy from the family plumbing business he had eventually declined to join.

His fingers spread to touch me everywhere except where I wanted them most. Mordecai wedged his lean hips between my thighs. His thrusts echoed the rhythm of the push and pull of his tongue in my mouth.

During the past few weeks, learning his body had become an adventure. My hands drifted beneath his arms, along his taut oblique muscles. At his waist I slipped free the button and eased the zipper over his erection. My body responded with a premature pull between my legs. Hard, hot flesh leapt between my hands. Mordecai groaned into my mouth before his lips wandered across my cheek to my ear.

"Trust me, Stephanie." He made this demand during foreplay to reassure me that he would honor my decision not to be penetrated by his sex.

His breath tickled my neck. I rolled his length between my palms and agreed to every act he suggested.

He pulled free of my grasp before his orgasm could erupt.

My body hovered painfully near climax when Mordecai stopped touching me. I cried out in distressed anticipation.

He smiled a feral smile at me. His breath pumped his chest while he cautiously zipped his pants, then rose to his feet. Gazing down at me, he said, "If you unsnap your bra and remove your trousers, I'll give you a delicious treat." He walked toward the kitchen without waiting to hear my answer.

* * *

Mordecai returned to find me frozen and holding my trousers in front of my naked lower body in the center of my sun room. My face must have reflected my fear because he tossed the roll of plastic wrap onto an accent table and hurried to my side.

He won the struggle for my trousers.

"If I strip, I'll take you hard and fast until you can't walk." He discarded my trousers then tangled his fingers in the coarse hair between my legs. One dry finger pushed inside me. The friction triggered ripples along the path to my womb. "Let me do this for you, Stephanie."

I jerked against the small penetration although my own wetness made it painless.

"Yes," I said.

Mordecai's free arm embraced my torso and lifted me off my feet. I barely kept the pleasure of his finger.

He arranged me on the loveseat with my legs spread—one leg along its back, the other with my foot on the floor. Mordecai slid his palm beneath my buttocks to position a double-layered length of plastic under my hips. My own moisture trickled over my skin. He released my hips and placed the remaining flap of material over my swollen sex and erect clit. The slick texture taunted my nerve endings. I gasped for breath when his thick finger pushed the barrier deep inside me. My muscles clenched around his attempted withdrawal.

"One minute more, Stephanie," he said as he removed his leather belt from its loops.

I didn't think I wanted him to bind or whip me no matter how playfully, but he only cinched the belt around my waist to hold the makeshift loincloth in place. He reached for my upper thighs with hands that trembled.

Mordecai stared between my legs until I fought his hold. He met my frantic expression with a baring of his teeth. "You look ripe to be plucked."

His thumbs peeled apart the petals of my sex. His head ducked toward my vulnerable core. I heard him murmur, "Discount wrap gives protection without eliminating the scent."

His mouth consumed me as if he feared he'd never again eat. When not reaching for my womb, his tongue made infrequent shallow stabs at the clenched opening between my buttocks.

Lying completely exposed in the daylight in a room with more windows than walls didn't concern me as much as my need for orgasm. My hands twisted his perfectly formed ears until he moved my hands to my breasts. The feel of my own sensitized flesh snapped my control.

I screamed my demands with profane simplicity.

Mordecai complied.

* * *

Dressed only in my trousers, I lay sprawled across his naked body on the floor. His fingers massaged the base of my spine.

"Unless you object, Stephanie Jeffers, I plan to have you as soon as possible after you introduce me to your family." He spoke in his professional voice, but smiled brilliantly when I glanced up at his face.

Regardless of the uncertainty of a future with Mordecai, I decided that I deserved to have my first experience of sexual intercourse with the man of my dreams.

"No objections, Mordecai Burk." His heart beat strong and steady beneath my ear.

"Full tilt after cocktails this Friday," he said.

* * *

"I replaced the leaky joint and repaired the small weak spot in the wall," Mordecai's oldest brother Alonzo said to me as he gathered his scattered tools. "Good thing Mordecai noticed the discoloration and recognized what it meant."

I followed him out of the main bath and down the stairs to the foyer where I offered him a signed check and a pen. "Just write in the amount, Alonzo."

He plucked the draft from my fingers and ripped it into fourths before pressing the pieces into my open palm. "Fix me a pot of that vegetarian chili and a loaf of that sweet bread you made for Mordecai last month and we're even."

During the tax rush I had provided large quantities of easy to heat meals as my contribution to helping Mordecai maximize productivity in his hectic work schedule.

"Deal."

Alonzo's beauty had been revealed to me slowly over the course of several months. Initially his patched eye and scars had distracted my vision. Now when I looked at him I saw a trustworthy friend and loving son, brother, and fiancé to Jessamine Winterberry. I knew him well enough to be concerned by his direct gaze as he lingered inside my front door.

"When Jessamine proposed marriage to me, I wondered if her big heart pitied me as something broken, someone only her love could fix." His eye traveled over my frowning face. "I stalled for months, thinking of myself as an honorable man giving her sufficient time to recognize her mistake." Alonzo smiled Mordecai's sheepish grin at me. "She won that standoff. She sees me and loves me for the whole man that I am." He hefted his tools under one brawny arm. He unlocked the door and opened it before he turned toward me again. "Jessamine loves me as much as my baby brother loves you. Good luck Friday. Call me when my food is ready. Bye."

He was inside his truck and backing into the street by the time my shock receded.

* * *

The first hour of cocktails and hors d'oeuvres at Mordecai's house passed very smoothly despite my sisters' unsanctioned decision to invite my parents. The six of us lounged in the comfortable furniture grouped around the fireplace in his music room. Various Duke

Ellington compositions cycled through the audio system and provided melodic accompaniment to my father's polite inquisition.

"Yes, Mr. Jeffers," Mordecai said in response to the most recent of the dozens of questions my father asked. "More than fifty percent of my clientele stayed with me when I left the firm."

As a tax accountant who served the needs of small businesses, Mordecai had been an independent consultant working out of his home for five years. I could see that my investment broker parents were impressed by the loyalty Mordecai inspired in his clients.

"Now it's time to consider taking on a partner before my client load overwhelms me."

My father asked for specific details about Mordecai's long-range personal and professional goals.

Mordecai graciously indulged my parents' old-fashioned need to know that their daughter was involved with a good provider. His smile and affable manner never slipped no matter how probing my father's questions became. My mother's and sisters' atypical reticence unnerved me. Their gazes shifted between

Mordecai and me, and scrutinized us from head to toe. Their smiles were identical harbingers of imminent mischief.

"Pardon me," Mordecai and I said. He grabbed the empty wine bottle in its cask while I escaped toward the powder room.

* * *

On my return to the music room I stepped into the central passage where all the first floor spaces opened.

"She showed you the photos?" My older sister Ashley's sultry voice floated from the kitchen. The low pitch of Mordecai's reply registered as only a positive murmur.

I leaned against the sueded wall and edged my way closer. Mordecai arranged finger foods on a tray. Ashley watched and occasionally pilfered a sample.

"Stephanie's photos revealed an adolescent with a severe case of acne, not the hideous monster she described." He paused and glanced in my direction as if he sensed my presence.

Ashley stood with her back to me. "She drank only water. Avoided junk food. Exercised religiously. Her allergic reactions to prescribed medications were as severe as the acne." Ashley's voice echoed with a protective sibling's sympathy and impotence. "Steph withdrew so much. All she did was study, and read for pleasure. Her only outside activities were her part-time job as proofreader for the community newsletter and volunteering to read for the blind."

In addition to understanding Ashley's motives, the fact that Mordecai already knew every detail Ashley had spoken kept me from feeling embarrassed or betrayed by her revelations even though her stark summary portrayed my high school years as pathetic.

Ashley propped her hip against the granite countertop. Shoulders back, she leaned toward Mordecai. Her body language warned me to brace myself to hear an outrageous statement.

"What are your intentions toward Stephanie?"

As much as I desired to hear Mordecai's answer, my fear and guilt were stronger. I quickly tiptoed to the music room where my parents and Antonia conspicuously stopped conversing when I entered.

Their identical bland smiles alerted me to prepare myself for the next phase of my family's well-meaning conspiracy.

* * *

The next hour passed like years of purgatory.

After the tour of Mordecai's home—requested simultaneously by my sisters—my father said, "You make a favorable first impression, Mordecai Burk. For your sake, it better be real." It was my father's conditional approval.

With a look I'd seen throughout my childhood, my mother conveyed her understanding of my hopes and fears. She and my sisters arranged themselves on either side of my father. Mordecai faced them, and I stood in the space between the two factions.

"Thank you, Mr. Jeffers." Mordecai's fingers snagged mine. "Stephanie and I will see you often enough for you to confirm that I am the man I appear to be."

My father smiled. When he extended his hand Mordecai completed the gesture. My mother and sisters thanked and hugged him. Their sly grins promised me a thorough interrogation within the next few days.

"We survived," Mordecai said as we waved my family down the street. He draped his arm around my shoulders and squeezed me. "Thank you for the honor of meeting your family, Stephanie."

I watched Mordecai's beautifully shaped free hand close the door, engage the locks, and set his alarm. He used his one-armed hold to pull me into a full-contact embrace.

He must have felt my tremors because he said, "No fear. No hurry, Stephanie. I will not hurt you." His fingertips tapped along the well of my spine. "I will not rush you." He angled his head until our gazes met. "Will you have me tonight, Stephanie?"

For the first time in my life I looked into the earnest face of a flesh and blood man and believed he desired me. My deepest fantasy manifested in reality.

"Yes," I said.

Mordecai bared his teeth and swung me into his arms.

* * *

Warm water drenched our bodies from four nozzles strategically spaced around the cylindrical stall. My soapy hands glided over Mordecai's neck and shoulders. From his kneeling position he leaned forward to taste the skin around and in my navel. His strong wet hands held the backs of my thighs and braced my legs apart while my hands savored the feel of his smooth muscular flesh. Bathing him was a luxury too precious to squander. I urged him to his feet with a tug on his ears.

Mordecai propped his hands on my hips and kissed his way from my waist to my breasts where he lingered over my distended nipples with his agile tongue. My palms caressed the tight skin over his breastbone in increasingly wider circles. My thumbs flicked his nipples on each pass. Mordecai remained silent, but my throaty sounds of sensual distress filled the enclosure.

Taking him inside of me became my only coherent thought.

When I would have reached for his erection, Mordecai snatched me into a crushing embrace that trapped my arms between our bodies.

In my ear he whispered, "I've been celibate for thirteen months; since the day you helped me gather spilled oranges from my driveway." One arm clamped across the base of my spine while the other hand turned the faucet. He told me he was free of STDs before he asked, "Are you?"

"Yes," I said as he stepped from the stall and held us in the stream of warm air flowing from the body dryer.

He carried me into his bedroom and laid me across the width of his bed. I supported myself against my elbows and watched him sheath himself in latex.

"Stephanie, for you I'd go bare, but it's too early in our relationship to consider pregnancy, right?"

Dazed, all I could do was nod. I collapsed against the luxurious texture of the Egyptian cotton duvet, and closed my eyes until Mordecai's body covered me. My eyes snapped open to find myself the center of his pensive regard.

His body heat warmed me. His lean hips settled between my thighs. Trepidation muted a small portion of my desire even as I placed my arms around his neck and smiled.

"Do you love me, Stephanie?"

My smile slipped. A truthful answer would make me vulnerable; expose me to ridicule. Ashley always reminded me that lack of courage resulted in no love. I wanted Mordecai's love.

"I love you, Mordecai Burk."

His smile blessed me. "Thank you, Stephanie." He gathered me into his arms and rolled until he reclined on his back and I rested atop his tightly strung body. "I love you, Stephanie Jeffers. You've claimed me moment by moment over the past year." He arranged my legs astride his hips.

The feel of his firm, hot erection pressed against my clit jolted me and started a roiling sensation in the pit of my stomach.

"Kiss me," he said.

* * *

"Please," I whispered against his lips before I pushed my tongue into his mouth.

Mordecai had teased and tantalized me until we both teetered at the verge of sexual meltdown.

We lay on our sides, face to face. His hand lifted my top leg and propped it over his hip. He wedged himself against the junction of my thighs. The engorged head of his penis slipped between my slick, swollen folds. Instantaneous orgasm swamped my body.

From a distance I heard Mordecai say, "Open your eyes, Stephanie."

By concentrating I managed to drag my eyelids half open. Mordecai's panting breaths caressed my face with puffs of air while he slowly pushed his thick, stiff length into my snug passage. His eyes narrowed as my body's resistance increased. Despite the lingering pleasure of orgasm, his presence brought me sharp discomfort.

His grasp on my hips tightened when he felt the thin membrane. Recognition, surprise, and pleasure flashed in his eyes. All my instincts clamored for me to expel his invading member. My muscles clamped around him. We groaned in unison.

"Thank you, Stephanie." Mordecai thrust hard and deep without pause. Seconds later his pubes met mine. "Thank you."

There was no pain, only a nearly unbearable fullness. I gasped for every breath. I had never felt so stretched, so possessed by and possessive of another person. Gradually my discomfort eased. Relinquishing my virginity had been different and much more than I had imagined it would be.

Mordecai correctly interpreted my smile as a prompt to continue my initiation.

A few slow thrusts and withdrawals spun us into ecstasy.

* * *

"Why not?"

By Saturday night the voice and manner of my indulgent lover were gone—replaced with those of an angry aggressor intent on achieving his goal.

"Renting my home and moving into yours is not a good idea. All our possessions would cram every available space."

Clad in Mordecai's pajamas and robes, we lounged in opposing wing chairs in the sitting area of his bedroom where I had allowed him to hold me captive for more than twenty-four hours. We ate from a tray of leftover hors d'oeuvres on the antique table between us. Mordecai glowered at me. I shoved a stuffed mushroom cap into my mouth.

"Stephanie, you love me. You trust me." He slid from his chair, moved aside the table, and knelt at my feet. "I'm your lover—your first, and if you're willing, your only lover for as long as I live."

Until he pulled the small jeweler's box from the pocket of his robe, I thought he was proposing informal, long-term cohabitation. I gulped my glass of wine.

"Choose me, Stephanie. In front of God, our families, and our friends, join our lives."

A solitary, round pink diamond sparkled from its Tiffany setting on a platinum filigree band. I looked from the ring to Mordecai's open expression, which revealed his love for me. The cacophony of my insecurities whispering in my ear faded. The ugly girl I had been so long ago encouraged me to accept the gifts Mordecai offered.

"Yes, Mordecai Burk, I'll marry you."

UNSPOKEN TRUTHS

The formal photograph showed a dark, handsome man and a darker, unbelievably beautiful woman seated upon an intricately carved bench. The couple gazed at each other with apparent devotion. Behind them, a lanky teenager stared directly into the lens with big, solemn eyes that overpowered his gaunt face. The ornately framed picture seemed misplaced in the airy informal setting of R.J. Bakerman's sunny home library. For the first time after months of visits I reached out to touch the haunting captured image.

"He used me as his whore for seven-hundred twelve days."

Previous conversations had taught me never to underestimate the reclusive novelist's penchant for calmly delivering shocking revelations. I turned to meet his impassive gaze. His man's body had grown into balance with the boy's eyes. He radiated power, and strength, and unspeakable sadness.

"And on day seven-thirteen?"

R.J. strolled across the room, then lowered himself into a suede chair. He waved me closer until he had to tilt his head to see my face. His travesty of a smile forecast an unpleasant answer.

"Mother took me to a private clinic. After surgery, she stayed with me through recovery, then enrolled me in boarding school. I never lived with them again."

He watched me closely, looking for signs of repulsion and disgust. There weren't any—at least not any directed toward him.

"Did she press charges against your father? Divorce him?"

"Reverend Phillip Strathmore was not my father, Georgette." R.J. closed his eyes and rested his head against the bolster. "My father, Mother's first husband, died of complications from hypertension when I was five. And no, she did not press charges or divorce him."

What could I offer this man other than my outrage, which wouldn't heal him from or make him forget those painful seven-hundred twelve days and their consequences?

"Why have you told me these things, R.J.?"

His short feathery lashes fluttered against his skin before his eyelids popped up.

"I hate being touched by people." His hand reached toward mine, then dropped back to the chair arm. "I want you to touch me," he whispered. "I dream about your touching me."

R.J. Bakerman was the most critically and commercially successful writer my firm, Very Fine Print Literary Agency, represented. His high-octane testosterone fiction always entered the best sellers' lists among the top three. I worried that intimate involvement with him might be counter-productive as well as unethical.

If my choice proved to be foolhardy, there were other agents or agencies I'd feel confident recommending.

I knelt to the side of his chair and covered his hand with mine. At first he tensed as though he anticipated pain. Minutes later, his entire body visibly relaxed. We sat with only our hands touching for more than an hour. We never discussed his most recent manuscript.

* * *

Following a pattern established during the weeks since R.J.'s revelation about his desire to be touched by me, we walked hand-in-hand around the perimeter of the small duck pond located near the southern edge of his hundred-acre property. It had been a thriving family-owned horse breeding concern until financial mismanagement and death forced the sale of the stock and land.

We walked in the silence we had maintained since our brief greeting at his front door thirty minutes earlier. Spring sun and breeze saturated and embraced us. Lush rough cushioned our bare feet. Deep breaths put the taste of grasses on my tongue. R.J.'s slow long-legged pace allowed me to stroll also. His fingers laced mine in a grip that did not bind. My palms were callous from summers of working in my family's plumbing business, but I was curious to know about the cause of his rough palms. Thinking about the touch of his hand started fantasies regarding other places I'd like him to touch, but my decision always to wait for him to initiate physical contact had served me well in the past weeks.

69

When R.J. slowed to a full stop, I stopped with him. He released my hand, stepped close behind me, and embraced me tightly with his arms looped around my shoulders. His bristly chin rubbed my temple. The pure, musky scent of him filled my chest while the ducks' squawking conversation drifted on the breeze. I sagged into his strong body trusting him to support my weight. His growing erection nudged my buttocks.

"Thank you, Georgette," he said into my ear after he kissed it.

Whether he was expressing gratitude for business, pleasure or both, I didn't know or particularly care beyond its significance for R.J.

I said nothing because I sensed he would tell me more in his own time. We stood watching the ducks against the distant backdrop of the trees that marked the southern boundary of his property. As the afternoon waned, the pond reflected the sun's intensity with weaker results.

R.J. said, "I enjoy your touch, Georgette."

Reaching up to cover his hands with mine, I caressed the backs of his fingers with a brush of gentle circular strokes. His erection grew and prodded the cleft between my buttocks. I rotated my backside over his groin as I lamented the fact that neither of us thought to bring a blanket or condoms.

R.J. loosened his hold enough to turn me toward him. Dark brown eyes gazed into my eyes with complete honesty and vulnerability. "Whatever you offer, Georgette, I will value." He dropped his hands away from my shoulders and took two long steps backward.

The openness of his face combined with the fitness of his body and the patina of his skin partially covered by denim shorts and golf shirt drew me closer to him on all levels of attraction.

"Will you accept kisses from me, R.J.?" I asked, stepping almost close enough to brush his chest with my breasts.

R.J. answered by leaning toward me until our lips made fragile contact. I leaned forward to increase the pressure. We kissed gently and chastely for several minutes with our mouths as our only point of physical connection even though sexual desire sparked brightly between us. I wanted him to feel safe to approach me with his desires, so I encouraged him with acceptance of every move his mouth made on mine.

His tongue entered my mouth at the same moment his hands clasped my waist and lifted me into alignment with him from mouth to pelvis. Two layers of denim and two layers of cotton knit prevented us from touching skin-to-skin where we most wanted to touch while his tongue thoroughly claimed every surface of my mouth.

R.J. lowered me to my feet and took his hands from my waist before he grabbed the hem of his shirt and tugged it over his head. It fell to the ground behind him while he reached for my shirttail and tugged it free of my waistband. In seconds I stood before him in denim shorts and a sheer white bra that revealed the dark skin of my breasts and the darker skin of my areolae and nipples. Under R.J.'s fixated stare my nipples grew tighter and puckered. My breasts throbbed with heaviness.

R.J. shook himself into motion. He gathered our shirts to spread them on the grass as a narrow blanket, then stepped to me and wrestled me out of my shorts and sheer panties as if I were struggling against him.

Wetness dampened his hand when he pressed the back of it between my legs. The other hand caressed the side of my face. He smiled at me. In this peaceful and sunny place, he gave me a smile free of sadness and doubt.

I lay on my back on the makeshift blanket without his asking. He knelt beside me to arrange my arms over my head. The sun and breeze heightened the agitation R.J. had started. His physical beauty and the sexual attraction between us jolted my pulse into a faster beat. I let my eyes convey my trust and desire for him.

He reclined on his side and slowly rolled atop me. I spread my legs. We jostled against each other to achieve a perfect fit. His hands joined mine above my head. The feel of him obscured my sense of all other stimuli. My slick folds rubbed against the worn denim of his shorts, which strained to hold his erection. My eyes stayed with his when he pressed his firm chest into my breasts. Feeling his smooth skin through the sheer barrier of my bra tweaked the link between my breasts and womb. I gasped for breath.

As if finally convinced of my compliance, R.J. closed his eyes and kissed me gently. His tongue enticed mine into his mouth where I soothed the warm, sweet cavern with quick sweeps of flesh and enamel. His mouth left mine to chart a path around my face, across my chin, and down my neck that tickled a laugh from me. The weight of him pinned me, preventing me from moving against him to soothe my need. His kisses moved over my skin in a slow dragging motion that increased my anticipation for his next move. He was silent in his homage to my body, but his body trembled atop my immobilized limbs.

He kissed the upper swells of my breasts, then skipped their mass and swirled his lips all over my abdomen. My sob of frustration stopped his progress and opened his eyes. He raised his head long enough to lave each of my nipples with his tongue before he returned to kissing my abdomen. Sheer fabric held the moisture while the fluttery breeze cooled it on my heated skin raising chill bumps.

R.J.'s downward course brought my hands near my hips, allowing me to arch my back in futile search of relief for the pressure building between my legs. R.J. released my hands to clasp my upper thighs and push my legs wide apart until my muscles quivered with the effort. I felt my vaginal muscles clenching prematurely in anticipation of being filled with some part of R.J.

He suckled the tender skin at the tops of my thighs, then licked into me deeply without any warning. His nose brushed the underside of my clit causing me to grab his head and grind his face between my legs while sensation skittered along my nerve endings. He must have expected my reaction because he only licked deeper in response. He lapped at me as if I were a feast presented to a man denied sustenance for years. His tongue worked me into a sudden, strong orgasm that doused his face.

While I lay sprawled, experiencing receding waves of orgasm, R.J. knelt between my spread legs and gingerly unfastened his shorts. His chest pumped like a bellows and his breath huffed from his open mouth. The head of his penis showed above the waistband of his briefs. He shoved down his garments, wiped my dew from his face with both hands, then wrapped his penis in all ten fingers. His firm glide and milk technique fascinated me as much as the rapturous expression on his face while his gaze alternated between my face, my sex, and all points between.

When I rose to my knees, R.J. frowned his disappointment until I reached forward to cup his heavy testicles in one hand. Two fingers of my other hand disappeared between the swollen folds of my labia.

* * *

Later, we lay naked with my body draped across his completely relaxed lean muscle mass. The rough pads of his fingers tapped a lover's code along my spine. Regardless of its duration, this affair would be good for both of us.

* * *

"If she's dating that novelist, why would she lie about it, Alonzo?" Mordecai asked, and Coridan underscored the question with a grunt.

The Burk brothers speculated about their sister's love life while they lounged in Coridan's sauna after an early morning row on the river.

"Why ask me when it's your wife who introduced them, Mordecai?" The steamy haze weakened the effect of Alonzo's hard glare at his youngest sibling. "What does Stephanie say?"

"She claims she knows nothing about it."

Coridan rolled up from his supine position along one bench. "His books are disturbing. All about betrayal, dishonor, and retribution. We need to meet him, but that won't happen if we harass Georgette. If there's anything to tell, she'll come to us when she's ready." Coridan was only one year older than Georgette. They had always been closer to each other than to their other siblings.

"What if this were Maya, Dan?"

Coridan shrugged. "My daughter is three years old. There're years to go before I need to worry about her driving out to some eccentric's isolated retreat every other day of the week. Georgette is an intelligent and wise woman. Trust her."

Alonzo and Mordecai grumbled in acknowledgement of the truth of their brother's words.

* * *

R.J. welcomed me with a gentle hug. My hands brushed across the muscular definition of his broad shoulders and back. He tolerated the pressure of my clasped hands at the base of his spine for a few seconds before he retreated deeper into the media den.

I squeezed in along his side in the comfortable chair we shared. Our bare feet played footsie on the tufted ottoman. His arms held me close. His cheek warmed my temple.

"Your verdict, Georgette?"

"It's a charming, bittersweet love story, R.J."

"But?"

"But, your readers will be expecting espionage and violence if you release this manuscript under your own name." I nuzzled my face against his neck and kissed the warm resilient flesh. He no longer jumped as if goosed when I casually touched him. "Would you be willing to create a pseudonym? Maybe arrange to include excerpts in the next releases by Lorene Cary, Benilde Little, Nicholas Sparks or similar writers?"

R.J. pulled me atop his body and spread my legs on either side of his hips. Cool air reached my naked bottom under the rising hem of my short jersey dress. Weeks earlier I'd started dressing in ways that eased access to R.J.'s touch. He stared into my eyes as he pulled the hem to my waist. His strong fingers gripped the backs of my thighs while his thumbs pressed into the soft resilience of my skin. I arched my back to press my clitoris and wet slit against the bulge trapped behind his trousers. He pulled my thighs farther apart, then filled his hands with my buttocks and squeezed.

"Since the time you walked away from me at the end of our first meeting, I've been fantasizing about the feel of you."

My buttocks had always been more sensitive to tactile stimuli than my breasts. The alternation between hard kneading, soft caresses, and stinging slaps brought me to a rigidly intense orgasm.

In the aftermath, R.J. rocked my weeping sex over his stiff erection. The pressure tormented my exposed bud. He finally tugged my dress up my torso and over my head. His smile grew as he scrutinized my nakedness. His hands framed my face, but his hips continued rocking me toward another orgasm.

"What do you want, Georgette?"

Suppressing imminent orgasm was difficult, but I managed to hold off and focus on his face.

"I want you naked, now, RJ." I grappled with his belt, shoved his cashmere sweater under his arms, and unfastened his trousers.

A nervous laugh escaped me when his latex sheathed erection saluted me as I worked his boxer shorts down his legs.

"You knew?" I asked.

"Hoped. Desired," he said.

He tossed off his sweater while I pulled his trousers and boxers down his legs. Finally, his body was naked, and mine to pleasure. I shoved away the ottoman to kneel between his knees.

"May I kiss you?" I asked.

RJ. pulled me into his embrace by clasping my shoulders and hauling me close. His kiss was a carnal invasion. His fingers tangled in the roots of my hair. His tongue licked my lips and filled my mouth. My hands splayed over his closely cropped hair. He held me immobile without hurting me. Infrequent tremors shook his body.

"How do you want to take me, Georgette?"

I rubbed my breasts over his well developed pectorals.

"However you want to be taken, R.J."

* * *

"Hey, Beautiful, go for a walk with your favorite brother."

My assistant had standing orders to admit members of my family without announcing them.

"Dan," I said without looking up from the documents on my desk. "Give me one minute. Have a seat."

The documents could wait, but I needed the time to recommit to my personal vow of silence regarding my affair with R.J. If Coridan's scouting mission precipitated a brotherly visit to R.J., my heart and my career would be in jeopardy.

My brother stood behind me and leaned over my shoulder.

"Alonzo and Mordecai are ready to invade Bakerman's property to get their answers since you can keep a secret for three lifetimes."

With Coridan it was best to divert him from his mission by appearing to be forthcoming with information.

"R.J. Bakerman is my agency's springboard into the publishing stratosphere. He's produced seven global bestsellers in the past ten years—three translated into blockbuster films." Coridan propped himself against the edge of my desk. My gaze held his without swerving. "Very Fine Print is now big time, Dan." Prior to R.J.'s signing with me, a productive group of mid-list authors had kept my agency's profit margin very comfortable.

"Come on, Georgie, no sins of omission between us. You're with Bakerman whenever you're not here or at the teen hotline office. You glow whenever you hear or say Bakerman's name." Coridan wrapped his fingers around my hand. "Is it love, Georgie?"

Coridan's tone of voice told me that the answer seemed obvious.

"It's complicated, Dan."

"Either he loves you or he doesn't. Which is true?"

None of my brothers would support my choices regarding R.J. if they knew the details, but Coridan would worry without hearing some kind of definitive statement from me.

"Right now, Bakerman and I share a need. Our relationship is mutually beneficial." I rose from my seat and hugged my brother for comfort and to hide from the skeptical expression on his face. "Thanks for caring. Let's walk."

* * *

R.J. handed the sealed pouch to the waiting courier. R.J. turned from the closed door, grabbed me under my arms, and spun me around until we were too dizzy to stand.

"Thank you, Georgette," he said as we collapsed into his decadent leather sofa. "Thank you."

Thomasina Bloodworth of Bloodworth and Peters Publishing had read R.J.'s new 500-page manuscript in a three-hour reading marathon that resulted in the negotiation of terms within 48 hours of my first call to her after she received R.J.'s novel.

"R.J., your storytelling talent earned you the contract you just signed. Thank you for trusting me to represent you."

His lips smiled against the side of my neck while his hands explored me from breasts to thighs.

"Let's celebrate our brilliance with a feast." His pelvis jerked against my pubic bone before he stood and pulled me onto my feet to stand in front of him. "You're the first course. Run. This is your head start."

I was already in the hall.

* * *

When he caught me I was dressed in a diaphanous shortie nightgown and leaning over the high platform bed to pull back the bed linens. The flat of his hand between my shoulders pushed me face forward into the mattress. His other hand reached between my legs. Two fingers thrust toward my womb. His dry thumb penetrated my virgin rear. His legs propped apart my knees until my toes barely touched the floor. The taboo penetration heightened the intensity of my vaginal orgasm.

The heavy cotton of his shirt abraded my back.

"Would you take a plug between these sweet cheeks," he wiggled his thumb, "to stretch you wide enough for an erect penis?"

The invasion of his fingers and thumb pushed me beyond pleasure.

"No." I gasped for every breath.

"Would you allow me to grab you by your hair, call you 'bitch,' and dry hump you until you bled; until you had chronic hemorrhoids?"

My orgasm hit fast and hard, and still R.J.'s hand plunged between my legs and buttocks.

"Answer me."

"No. No. No," I answered to the rhythm of the push and pull of his fingers.

R.J. collapsed atop me, which shoved his digits deep inside me forward and rear.

"Then why did I?" he asked just before I slumped beneath his weight as my orgasm receded.

* * *

"You were a child," I said.

R.J. watched me unbutton his shirt, unbuckle his belt, and loosen his trousers. His feet were bare. "Your mother's husband betrayed you; abused his power as a parent; betrayed his position as an authority figure in the community."

R.J. raised his arms and his hips whenever necessary to help me undress him. "He made you feel responsible for his crimes against you. He stole your right to be safe in your own home, in your own body."

We were both naked. R.J. watched me as if he wanted to believe my words, but some part of his mind doubted his own innocence.

"Did he ever give you pleasure, R.J.?"

He didn't close his eyes fast enough to hide their sudden watery sheen. He shook his head. "Only pain, fear, and shame." R.J. slid under the sheets and rolled away from me. "Enough shame to kill me, Georgette."

He flinched when I stroked his arm. I snuggled the front of my body against his back and draped my arm around his waist.

"It is not your shame, R.J."

His fingers laced with mine over his rippled abdomen. Salty moisture wet my lips when I kissed the side of his jaw.

"May I give you pleasure, R.J.? You are worthy of pleasure. Will you accept it from me?"

His utter lack of movement alarmed me. What if my offer increased his sense of shame? I was guessing that feelings of unworthiness kept him isolated from people as much as the location and acreage of his home. The unconscionable acts of one man had forced R.J. to hide his intelligence, talent, and physical beauty. I wanted him to live every moment fully and free of past hurts, but what did R.J. want for himself?

R.J. rolled until I lay pinned beneath his warm, heavy body. His eyes watched me with trepidation and hope. "Pleasure me, Georgette."

Tears drenched my cheeks even though I smiled. I wrapped my arms around his neck.

The pleasuring began.

* * *

Two weeks later, I gloated over the fact that R.J. had agreed to meet me downtown for a lunch meeting with Thomasina Bloodworth. The risks of his being recognized were slim because his book jackets showed only charcoal sketches of his three-quarter profile.

My assistant slipped into my office and closed the door behind her.

"Georgette, Rev. Phillip Strathmore and Mrs. Jeanie Strathmore are here to see you. They just arrived from Atlanta. They want to discuss a private matter. You need to leave in thirty minutes."

After a brief moment of denial, I thanked whatever spirits had helped me to convince R.J. to meet me at the restaurant instead of at my office.

"Send them in, Lisa, then take off the rest of the day. Enjoy yourself. See you tomorrow."

In the next minute, two people of average height and extraordinary physical beauty entered my office. The photograph I had studied so many times had magnified their stature and diminished their beauty. I realized that Phillip Strathmore appeared larger in the photograph because R.J. was so young and small in the background.

After introductions, Phillip Strathmore said, "Rudyard's former agent gave us your direction—" He inspected my left hand. "—Miss Burk. Your client, R.J. Bakerman, is legally known as Rudyard James Strathmore. I adopted him when he was seven."

His voice was as smooth and rich as his complexion. None of his external features marked him as a rapist. Nothing about Mrs. Strathmore's appearance suggested that she would exile her child from his home rather than publicly accuse the monster she married.

Remnants of my breakfast churned in my stomach. I had nothing kind or mature to say to these people.

"If you had contacted me before making this trip, I would have told you that I'm not at liberty to discuss my clients beyond information pertaining to my duties as their literary representative." I rose from my chair. "Good day. I'm on my way out."

Mrs. Strathmore removed an envelope from her handbag. Her husband's eyes widened and tracked the progress of the buff colored six-by-nine rectangle from his wife's purse to my hand. "Please, Miss Burk, please give this to my son. Tell him—"

A door opened in the outer office. Only Lisa, R.J., and I had keys to my office. I begged any listening spirits to make Lisa the person who would walk through my door in the next three seconds.

"Georgette?" A flowering plant filled the widening gap as the door opened behind the Strathmores. "Let's ride in together, then catch a show or visit a gallery after—" R.J.'s arms tightened around the base of the potted plant. His back thumped the door jamb. For an instant his eyes accused me of betrayal. I slipped the envelope beneath the desk blotter.

"Don't your parents deserve a greeting, Rudyard?" Phillip Strathmore's bravado didn't make him fool enough to step closer to R.J.

Mrs.Strathmore swayed on her feet. My first priority was to protect R.J. I stepped closer to the woman; put my arm around her shoulders to keep her from moving closer to R.J.

"The Strathmores just arrived and are on their way out because I couldn't provide them with any information, R.J." He watched my lips as if he could not hear my voice. "If the plant's for me, thank you and put it on that shelf." I tipped my head toward the farthest corner of the room.

R.J. never turned his back on the Strathmores. He watched them with absolute concentration while he backed toward the shelf.

"We should not have come, Phillip. It's time to leave." Mrs. Strathmore touched her husband's arm.

"Not until he speaks to us, Jeanie. We raised him to act civilized."

R.J. twisted from the waist to set the plant on the shelf. His empty hands flexed and relaxed several times. Slowly, R.J. approached Phillip Strathmore who extended his hand, but lowered it when R.J. waved it away like fanning noxious fumes. R.J.'s fist landed squarely on his mother's husband's cheek. Strathmore swayed wildly, but didn't fall.

"You raped me."

Phillip Strathmore inhaled deeply. One hand cupped his cheek. His nostrils flared. His eyes narrowed.

R.J. continued in a severely modulated tone. "Your piety and respectability are smoke and mirrors that lure and deceive. I wasn't the first child you destroyed, but I pray that I was the last. I believe the universe is just, so I will not hate you or curse you. Never contact me again."

R.J. stepped around his mother's husband and spoke to Jeanie Strathmore. "If Georgette agrees, you may send correspondence to me here, care of Ms. Burk." No hint of emotion warmed his voice.

Mrs. Strathmore smiled. "Thank you. You've made yourself into a very fine human being. Somewhere your father is bursting with pride over you." She ended our side-by-side embrace with a quick squeeze of my waist before she claimed her husband's arm.

The couple departed quietly.

As soon as the outer door clicked shut and locked automatically, R.J. dropped to his knees and wound his arms around my waist.

"I fought him. He can't hurt me."

R.J.'s body trembled as if palsied. He broke into a sweat that saturated his clothes and mine.

Thomasina Bloodworth called to delay our meeting by one hour.

* * *

To R.J. Bakerman,

Although I think of you as my beloved child,
I will not address you as such because I abdicated
my parental privileges the day I consciously chose
to ignore the signs that my husband's interest in
you threatened every aspect of your well-being.

This is not a request for forgiveness.

Upon my return from enrolling you into boarding
school, I became my husband's keeper to ensure that
he harmed no other children. A year after you
terminated all communication with us, we traveled
to Africa to participate in a three-month mission.
My vigilance waned. My husband raped one of the
children in the host village. The child's mother
castrated Phillip, who nearly died from infection.
Mission administrators expedited our return to the
U.S. The board of directors at my husband's church
encouraged him to resign his position as pastor,
which is the primary reason we now live in Atlanta
where we support ourselves through our seedling

> enterprise and his inheritance. I give you these
> details only to reassure you that Phillip has no
> unsupervised interaction with potential victims.
> You deserve to know.
> I love you, RJ. My past failures to protect
> you give you valid reasons to doubt the veracity
> of my declaration, but it has always been true.
> Your books are mesmerizing and triumphant with
> endings so double-edged that they sometimes leave me
> feeling melancholy for days after reading them.
> Despite my criminal neglect and my husband's evil
> acts against you, you've become someone full of
> wonder. Be proud of the person you are, and every
> moment that brought you into being. You have earned
> peace of mind and happiness.

> *Jeanie*

His mother's letter had remained hidden under my desk blotter for three days. It took me another two days to decide to give it to RJ. Hearing her words of remorse and encouragement in RJ.'s voice made me glad that I had not returned the letter to her.

R.J. held the sheets of handmade, scented stationery in one hand while the other massaged his brow. Late afternoon sun passed through his French doors and gilded him in a chess pattern of light and shadow.

"She makes it difficult to hold a grudge." The sheets fluttered to the hardwood floor. R.J. escaped onto the deck where he paced its length several times. His stride suggested extreme agitation.

I went to the kitchen to start dinner.

* * *

R.J. fitted his body against my back as I finished removing the sauce pan from the burner and extinguished the flame. His hands fondled my breasts before he spun me face to face with him. My shirt fell away with the help of his dexterous fingers. R.J. spread my legs over either side of his thigh, palmed my buttocks in his hands, and bent to suckle strongly at my unbound breasts.

My primal scream did not distract R.J. from his mission to drive me into orgasm, as if controlling me would compensate for lack of control of his complicated feelings for his mother. Regardless of his motive, I trusted him not to hurt me. With my hands gripping the edge of the countertop and my body arched and thrusting against his, I abandoned myself to the immense pleasure.

R.J.'s sudden withdrawal left me teetering painfully near climax. His image swam in front of my eyes. A wet area showed on his pant leg.

He loosened his belt, stripped off his shirt, and pulled packaged latex from his pocket before he unzipped his fly. "Turn around and bend over, Georgette." His stance dared me to risk being sodomized.

I turned and bent over the counter. I fought the urge to clench my buttocks when R.J.'s hands braced apart my thighs after bunching my skirt around my waist. His fingers dipped into my overflowing sex, spreading my personal honey around and inside my puckered orifice. I moaned with each thrust of his big finger. He leaned on my back until my breasts were flattened against smooth, cold marble. My feet came off the floor. Fingers prized apart my cheeks, but the head of his penis slipped between my nether lips. With one steady stroke my rear and my sex were deeply penetrated. Pubic hair and the teeth of his open zipper tickled my skin when he rotated his hips. My passage squeezed around him in search of relief.

I used one hand to ease the pressure of the counter against my stomach. I satisfied my neglected clitoris with the shaky fingers of my other hand while R.J. applied steady pressure. His finger slipped free of my anus just before the heat and weight of his body blanketed my back, nudging his penis as deeply as I could take it. He pulled my hand away from my little erection. R.J. grasped my shoulders with an underhanded hold, bent his knees, and forced his way infinitesimally deeper. My distress escaped me in a high-pitched, keening wail. He held me spitted over him until my body more easily accommodated the depth of his presence.

Without loosing his tight grip on my shoulders, his hips moved forward and back with a small flex of his pelvis. My instantaneous orgasm left me feeling slightly nauseated.

By the time my equilibrium returned, my hands were braced against the counter while R.J.'s resolute grasp on my hips held me in place for the furious thrust and withdrawal of his penis as he achieved orgasm. He stiffened after one last, hard thrust, shuddered, and collapsed against my back.

* * *

"How can you trust me, Georgette? How can you love me so completely?" R.J. asked from somewhere close behind me.

I froze in the process of hand washing my silk nightie at one of the basins in the master bath. Throughout our affair I had intentionally avoided making verbal declarations of love because I feared the consequences of his response for both of us. I stared at the berry-colored garment that spent more time on the floor than on my body. I decided to risk everything.

My gaze collided with his in the framed mirror.

"Because you love me, R.J."

Every feature of his face contributed to his glorious smile. I spun to face him and we embraced like long-lost friends. My soapy hands wet the back of his shirt. We laughed into each other's faces. I thanked my parents and brothers for teaching me how to recognize love even when the words weren't spoken.

NAME GAME

He lay naked across the bed stripped down to its fitted sheet because he hated loose bed linens to interfere with his access to my body. His predatory smile enticed me to move from my position at the foot of the bed. Kneeling at the edge of the mattress between his spread legs, I placed my hands on his ankles and pressed his feet until his heels met the lower curves of his taut buttocks. My hands kneaded and slapped his turgid flesh and drawn sac while his hands gripped the thick spindles of the heirloom headboard. Latex stretched to accommodate the girth of his sex before my wet sheath did the same. Slowly, I rocked myself in the cradle of his legs. My body required a full minute to take him. His hands released the furniture in favor of a firm grip on my thighs, which he eased farther apart, compelling me to take him deeper by increments. The pungent smell of male and female arousal filled my nostrils and throat as full as his flesh filled my body. I needed to ride him hard, but he held me immobile. I gazed at him and saw my need reflected in his eyes.

"Kiss me," he said.

When I leaned forward, my clitoris pressed against his pelvic bone, jolting my nerve endings. I jerked against his restraining hold.

* * *

The first ring awakened me instantly.

"Hello, this is Dr. Kalliope Cleary Ruskin," I said feeling jittery from days of insufficient sleep.

A quick glance at the illuminated clock face confirmed that I'd been asleep for fewer than three hours. Dawn was about two hours away.

"Mommy, this Maya Burk. Daddy very hot. Please come now."

Hearing the sweet soprano voice of my former lover's four-year-old child brought a smile to my face until all her words registered. She usually called me "Dr. K" unless she was uneasy.

"Maya, let me speak to your daddy, please."

Cupcake, my two-year-old mostly shepherd mutt, barked once in recognition of the child's name.

"He won't talk." The frequency of the tremor in her voice suggested that fear rather than unhappiness gripped her.

"Maya, sweetheart, tell me why you're out of bed. Have a bad dream?" While the little girl gave details about calling for her daddy to chase away the bad man, I groped the surface of my bedside table for my wireless phone and dialed for emergency assistance.

"...He always comes right away, but he didn't come, Mommy." She hiccoughed.

"I understand, Maya, just hold on while I tell some people how to get to your house to help your daddy and you. Stay on the phone with me, Maya. Okay?"

" 'Kay."

Maya's heavy breathing and occasional sniffles sounded in one ear and the emergency dispatcher's voice sounded in the other while I slipped my feet into clogs and abandoned the idea of a robe or jacket because donning either garment would require me to relinquish either the cordless phone or the wireless. The dispatcher believed my summary of the situation, agreed to dispatch an ambulance to the address my memory hadn't purged, and disconnected our call in under ninety seconds. My mad dash through the house shortened my breath.

"Maya?" I said into the cordless.

Cupcake barked once, softly.

"Yes?"

"Sweetheart, I'm coming to your house right now. So is the ambulance. Don't get scared of the lights and sirens. They're coming to help you and your daddy. All right, Maya?"

Cupcake whined and circled my legs.

"All right, Mommy."

With keys and wireless phone in the patch pockets of my pajama top, I stepped from the kitchen to the garage and double-checked my medical bag in the trunk of my car. I needed to connect with Maya on my wireless phone to stay linked with her while I drove. Inside the car I'd be able to voice activate the speaker feature of my wireless system.

"Maya, are you in your daddy's bedroom?" The ignition caught while the garage door completed its ascent. Cupcake jumped into the open driver's door, wiggled into the back seat, then turned to me with his traveling harness in his mouth. There wasn't time to put him inside the house.

"Yes." Her little whisper made me think that she was looking at her father, whose appearance scared her.

Just over a year of monogamously dating Coridan Burk had granted me the privilege of knowing his home very well.

"Maya, walk into the next room where Daddy's books and desk are. When the phone on top of his desk rings, answer it. You'll hear my voice. Okay?"

We had ceased dating two months earlier, but his private and business numbers were still programmed into my wireless phone. I offed the cordless as soon as Maya's voice greeted me through the wireless.

Five minutes later, the ambulance and I arrived from opposite directions in front of Coridan's house.

* * *

Coridan's siblings and in-laws descended on the waiting room en masse. The cacophony of their arrival awakened Maya who had been sleeping sprawled across my lap. Everyone except Alonzo Burk wore some type of sleeping attire. They quieted to hear my summary of the physician's last briefing fifteen minutes earlier.

Maya's little arms and soft hands reached for her father's oldest brother. "Uncle Awonzo, Daddy feels very bad."

"I know, Maya." Alonzo lifted his niece into the crook of one of his brawny arms. "What a smart girl you were to call Dr. K," he said to Maya although his one-eyed gaze studied me.

The little girl smiled at someone behind her uncle. "Georgie!"

Georgette Burk and R.J. Bakerman took turns kissing and caressing the little heroine.

Mordecai Burk and Stephanie Jeffers, his wife, dropped into chairs on either side of me.

"Thank you, Kalliope," the couple said in unison.

The three of us shared a laugh. I'd missed seeing the Burk siblings and their mates during the two months since my breakup with Coridan, who still allowed Maya to participate in the monthly trips my pediatric medical practice sponsored to visit patients at the Children's Hospice.

"You're welcome."

When I asked about Ezechiel and Odessa Burk, Mordecai said, "The Parents are visiting relatives on the west coast. We decided not to alert them until we had details even though Mom always senses when one of us needs her." He looked toward the corner where Alonzo handed Maya into Jessamine's arms. "Looks like Big Brother is on his way to make the call now."

I wondered if news of Coridan's severe allergic reaction to tainted seafood would prompt the Burk family's matriarch and patriarch to return home immediately.

The attending physician had informed us that more than two dozen people who had dined at *Prince's Seaside Inn* the previous evening were admitted to various area hospitals. Coridan's case appeared to be the most extreme of those reported.

A nurse entered and waited for us to gather around her before she said, "Mr. Burk is in room C5. You may visit him in pairs for three minutes each pair before you go home. Come back later today during visiting hours. Understand?"

Alonzo stepped into the room as we all nodded our agreement to her dictates.

"Maya?" the nurse said. "Why don't you visit your father first since he keeps asking about you." The nurse's mellow voice and bright smile didn't fool my discerning ears and eyes: Coridan's concern for his daughter must be impeding the staff's ability to administer treatment, otherwise the four-year-old child would have been barred from visiting his room.

Jessamine exchanged a look with her husband Alonzo, who said, "Kalliope, would you take Maya in to see her dad?"

During my stunned silence, Jessamine turned toward me and Maya leapt from her aunt's arms to mine. Reflex opened my arms and caught her close to my chest. Her arms hugged my neck. She yawned, then smiled at me.

"Let's see Daddy, Dr. K."

This family's ability to act quickly and decisively as a group with unified intent had always impressed me. Now it unnerved me. They had implicitly agreed on a conspiracy to matchmake. I had no idea what, if anything, Coridan had said to his family about the reasons for our breakup.

"Please, Kalliope? You can explain whatever equipment is in the room to help Coridan," Mordecai said.

R.J. said, "One of us can take Maya to see Coridan, Kalliope. You're free to do what's best for you." Typically, he refused to witness manipulation—no matter how lovingly intended—without offering an escape.

The nurse seemed content to wait for my decision along with everyone else. I watched Georgette's fingers stroke the inside of R.J.'s wrist. The longer she touched him, the more tension seeped from his body until his stance relaxed completely.

The Burks had maneuvered me into position very handily, but their goal and mine were the same—to see Coridan.

"Thank you, R.J." I shifted Maya higher in my embrace. "Maya and I will see Coridan now, if everyone agrees."

The nurse led our solemn procession to Coridan's private room.

* * *

Even with wires and tubes trailing from his body, Coridan's appearance was healthier than it had been hours earlier.

"Don't talk," I said when he opened his eyes. Maya and I settled into the chair next to his bed. "Maya's here to kiss you goodnight, then we're off to bed. We'll see you later today during visiting hours." I placed my hand over his. "Squeeze once if you agree." His strong grip encouraged my hopes for his recovery.

"You scared me, Daddy." The surgical mask covered her face from her nose to her chin. Maya wiggled closer to Coridan. Her kiss smacked him right between the eyes. "You couldn't chase away the bad man because you was sick. Feel better, Daddy?" She balanced herself between the edge of the bed and my lap.

"Thanks to you, Maya, Daddy feels much better. You did everything right." The short statement seemed to drain his available energy. He closed his eyes.

"Alonzo, Jessamine, Georgette, R.J., Mordecai, and Stephanie are waiting to see you. Okay?" This time his single squeeze was noticeably weaker. "Your parents' flight arrives this afternoon. Less than fifteen minutes until peace and quiet."

Coridan smiled without opening his eyes.

* * *

Twenty minutes later it was obvious that the Burks had used their time waiting in order to coordinate their plan of action.

"Would you stay with Maya until Coridan's discharged day after tomorrow, Kalliope? You did say you left Cupcake in their backyard," Mordecai said, then looked to Alonzo for support.

"Or take Maya to your house since the General is away on a tour of the Holy Lands with her Ladies' Church Auxiliary. She returns in two weeks," Alonzo explained the whereabouts of Coridan's formidable live-in housekeeper, Mrs. Hannah.

Georgette Burk read the look of indecision on my face. She said, "It's no problem for me to stay with Maya. We just thought you two might enjoy some girl time with each other."

These people dangled the perfect lure. Other than two hospice excursions and one unscheduled office visit prompted by a minor asthma episode, I hadn't seen Maya since my breakup with Coridan. Today was the first of three scheduled consecutive vacation days for me. My two medical partners would probably agree to answer any emergency calls from my patients since I'd been on-call every weekend during the past two months.

Maya's sleeping body rested like a small, loosely packed bundle in my arms. She drooled on my shoulder.

"Cupcake and I will stay with Maya at her house so she'll be surrounded by the familiar."

The Burks nodded their agreement and smiled in celebration of their victory.

* * *

Maya and I slept until late afternoon. After a quick stretch workout in Coridan's home fitness studio, we bathed, dressed, and ordered a veggie pizza without cheese.

Cupcake barked repeatedly when a loud knock sounded at the front door. Maya ran ahead of me to the door while I counted bills and calculated a tip.

"Where's your key, Daddy?" I heard Maya shout at the bolted door as I approached.

Minutes later, the taxi driver was paid, the pizza was delivered, and an exhausted Coridan was reclining on a couch in the living room. Maya lay between the back support and his torso.

"None of your family called to say you were discharged earlier than expected, Coridan," I said softly from my kneeling position on the floor.

He didn't answer, but the way his eyes catalogued my attire of one of his linen shirts and a pair of his drawstring shorts made it obvious that he'd noticed my lack of a bra.

"Coridan?"

He dragged his gaze up to my eyes. "I opted out of another day of observation. An additional 24 hours of meds and rest, and I'll be better than new."

He was right: His color appeared healthy despite the obvious exhaustion caused by the twenty-minute cab ride from the hospital to home.

"Will you stay, Kalliope, for the next two days? Maya and I need you and want you to stay." Coridan watched me steadily. His gaze revealed nothing while I was sure mine revealed every facet of my fear and hope for what these days together might mean for all of us.

"I'll stay."

Coridan smiled.

Maya gingerly scooted over his body and hopped to the floor. She hugged my neck and kissed my cheek before she said, "Good! May we eat now, Dr. K?"

* * *

Coridan slept for fifteen hours. By the time he awoke, I had returned from taking Maya to Montessori school and making a quick stop by my home for clothes and toiletries.

"You kept my house key," Coridan said as I stepped into the foyer.

"You told me to keep it in case I came to my senses." That statement had been among the nicer ones said to me during our final argument.

Coridan took the overnight luggage hanging from my shoulder. "Sharing my wardrobe with you didn't bother me, Kalliope." He led the way to the guest room before I could respond.

Once inside the room, Coridan reclined on the bed while I unpacked my bag.

"Is changing your name too high a cost for us to be a family, Kalliope?"

I continued unpacking, then stored my luggage on a shelf in the closet. Coridan lounged with his arms folded beneath his head and his legs crossed at the ankles. Plump pillows supported his back. His beauty appealed to me as much as it ever had.

His posture didn't fool me: He wanted a fight.

"Is your pride worth the loss of our relationship, Coridan?"

Finally, he allowed me a glimpse of the storm that had been brewing in his mind for months.

"I love you. I want to marry you." He sat forward and swung his legs over the side of the mattress. "Maya wants us to be together. My family adores you. What more do you want, Kalliope?" Frustration and bewilderment echoed in his voice.

114

Twice, Coridan proposed marriage to me. After my first acceptance we engaged in lengthy, uninhibited sex that left me feeling tender and sated until Coridan whispered, "How soon do you want to become Dr. Kalliope Ruskin Burk?"

When I said, "I'll still be Dr. Kalliope Cleary Ruskin after we marry," we had our first gloves-off fight, which ended when I stripped off the black opal and diamond engagement ring, gathered my clothes, and fled.

The outcome of the second proposal had been very similar.

Coridan embodied every characteristic I desired in a mate; everything I desired to be to someone special. Not for the first time, seeing him made me re-examine my need to keep my name. I walked closer to him, knelt at his feet, placed my hands on his thighs, and looked up into his beloved face.

"You are Coridan Burk, but what if tomorrow you became Coridan Ruskin? How would that change affect your standing as the president and CEO of Burk Family Enterprises?"

The muscles beneath my palms flexed. His warm, fragrant breath caressed my face.

"How would people treat you? What would they expect from you as Coridan Ruskin? What would you expect from yourself?"

His gaze revealed such deep hurt to me. "You're comparing apples and eggplants, Kalliope."

"Your name reflects your identity. Mine does, too. 'Kalliope Cleary Ruskin' reflects my personal heritage and represents my medical pedigree and professional achievement. Relinquishing my name—even for the joy of having you for a husband—would devastate me in more ways than one, which is why my mother kept her name after marriage."

Coridan grasped me under my arms and lifted me into his embrace, rolling me onto my back and leaning over me. "Is this all about my misplaced *machismo* or does your being adopted play some part in this discussion?"

At thirteen years of age, Myna Johnson had given birth to me as a result of being raped by a neighborhood bully. Early in her pregnancy Myna and Dr. Ann Marie Cleary met each other in the ladies' room of the church they both regularly attended. My mother had listened while Myna tossed up her breakfast, then cried until my mother jimmied the lock on the stall and gathered the heartbroken girl into her arms where Myna felt safe enough to reveal the details of her situation. That encounter led to my being adopted at birth by Drs. Calvin Ruskin and Ann Marie Cleary, who discovered during their first year of marriage that pregnancy put my mother's life in extreme jeopardy. After one miscarriage and several medical opinions, my father decided to have a vasectomy.

Coridan knew the complicated circumstances of my family connections. Maybe my being adopted made me more sensitive about issues concerning identity, but I'd feel attached to my name even if my parents were my biological parents.

"Coridan, the way I feel about my name isn't going to change, regardless of the reasons why."

He leaned in close until his nose rubbed mine. He smelled clean, natural, and very familiar. The warmth of his nearness lulled me into believing we would create a way to be together. His lips pressed soft kisses across my face. My initial response to his sensual touch was the same despite the two-month drought: My mind dreamed and my body opened.

"Do you believe that I love you, Kalliope?"

I snapped into full consciousness. When I opened my eyes, his gaze held mine with its steady regard.

"Yes, I recognize your love for me, Coridan, just as you recognize mine for you." He released me when I twisted in his arms. I straightened my clothes and brushed my hair back from my face while he propped himself against the headboard. I sat cross-legged near the foot of the bed. "Maybe the surname conflict is a smoke screen obscuring more significant obstacles to our getting married. Maybe—"

Coridan chopped the air with his hand. "Maybe nothing, Kalliope. What if we adopted more children? What would their last name be? Burk or Ruskin?"

He knew that severe endometriosis made it highly unlikely that I'd ever conceive a child.

"Maya is enough for me, Coridan, but if we added children to our family, they could be Burk hyphen Ruskin or Ruskin hyphen Burk or Burk or whichever name the children prefer if they're old enough to choose."

A glimpse at the time had me rearranging the importance of the errands I needed to run before I picked up Maya from school. Coridan reached for me when I jumped off the bed. "I promised Maya buckwheat waffles and baked apples for dinner." His hand snagged my blouse, tugging me to a slow standstill yards from the bedroom door.

Slowly, Coridan rolled from the bed without releasing my garment. He looked down at me until I raised my face to his. "I'll consider all that you've said, Kalliope. Leave your list so I can order groceries to be delivered while you get Maya."

When we parted ways in the hall I was grateful for the reprieve.

Two days later we resumed our monogamous relationship.

* * *

"When's the wedding?" Jessamine asked me after I settled into the booth.

With one quick nod, Stephanie discouraged her sister-in-law's frontal attack. To me, she said, "Order your drink before the interrogation begins, Kalliope."

Georgette greeted me with her luminous smile, then handed me her menu. The three sisters-in-law chatted with each other, but I felt their eyes on me more than once.

Our server came and went. I looked at Jessamine, Stephanie, and Georgette. Our bimonthly lunch gatherings reminded me of my good fortune in having them as friends.

"Coridan hasn't proposed."

"Yet," Jessamine said.

Stephanie hushed her with a wave of her hand, then said, "Kalliope, your relationship with Coridan is none of our business. Of course we want to know details, but we love you both and think you two are happiest when you're with each other. So the topic of conversation is your choice."

Stephanie and I had met each other in a yoga class, and through her I met Georgette and Jessamine. She had also referred Coridan to me when he became displeased with Maya's pediatrician.

"Coridan needs to reconcile himself to the fact that I intend to be known as 'Dr. Kalliope Cleary Ruskin' regardless of my marital status. In the meantime,

Georgette has agreed to keep Maya and Cupcake so we can go to New Orleans for a few days."

"Georgie!" Jessamine gave her sister-in-law a playful nudge. "You let us sit here and speculate about their relationship when you had the insider's track. Shame on you." Jessamine's throaty laughter was contagious.

"I knew Kalliope would tell you what she wanted you to know." Georgette's typical serenity had deepened during her involvement with R.J. Bakerman. "But now that she's mentioned that the name thing is their major obstacle, I'll say this. It would be foolish for Coridan to lose you over a name. My brother is seldom foolish."

Stephanie said, "Even Mordecai, who's willing to accept unconventional practices, needed some time to make peace with my keeping my name. There are a few friends and relatives who still take issue with my decision, and we've been married for two years." Her hand covered mine on the tabletop. "Have faith, Kalliope."

Jessamine endorsed that advice with a fierce nod, then said, "And if that brother-in-law of mine uses me as an example, remind him that I switched from

Winterberry to Burk to lose three syllables and rise twenty-one slots in the alphabet."

We discussed innocuous subjects while our food was served.

As soon as our privacy was restored, Jessamine said, "When do you leave for New Orleans?"

We lingered over our lunch for two glorious hours of affirmation.

* * *

Music and voices and heady aromas from the constant stream of humanity in the French quarter drifted into the open doors of the balcony. Heavy, warm air filled my lungs. Coridan filled my body.

He lay solid and still beneath me. I turned my face into his chest to inhale his unique scent. My tongue flicked one nipple, then the other. The salt and sweat of him saturated my taste buds. Coridan dragged his hands from my waist to my hair, which he twined around his fingers and tugged until my eyes met his. His smile lured me closer. My closed lips pressed his before I brushed them back and forth from one corner of his mouth to the other. His erection swelled inside me.

Coridan turned aside his head. His breath tickled my ear. "My brother Mordecai asked me to imagine the next year of my life without you in it." A small pelvic tilt nudged my swollen clitoris against the hard foundation of his groin. After a long, guttural moan, he said, "I desire you to be in my life more than my pride needs you to change your name to Burk, Kalliope."

My vaginal muscles squeezed him tightly. Coridan's strong hands pulled at my knees until I knelt astride his firm hips. His hard thighs sloped behind me. Each jostling of our bodies pushed me closer to orgasm. Coridan handled my passive limbs with gentle intent. Seconds later his thighs supported my back and his chest flattened mine while his tongue plundered my mouth and his hands pressed my hips, deepening his already deep penetration. My fingernails raked his shoulders as I came hard and fast. His tongue swept my mouth when I opened it wide to keen my pleasure. Coridan's short jabbing thrusts drove me toward another crest before I'd recovered from the previous orgasm.

His kiss moved from my mouth to my breast with little nips along the way. He suckled one breast while his left hand squeezed the other breast and tormented its nipple. His right hand caressed its way over my ribs and abdomen to brush cross my mons. His fingers tugged the tightly coiled curls before his knuckles pressed hard against the sensitive layer of fat. Coridan's arms blocked my hands away from my clitoris. I climaxed while we struggled.

Coridan's hands caught my wrists and held my arms spread wide. He gave me one warning glance before he resumed suckling my breasts. My body trembled from excessive stimulation. With my head still spinning from multiple orgasms, my body prepared for another.

Coridan twisted to one side, dropped me onto my back, and followed me down without dislodging his body from mine. He bent my arms, folding my hands on top of my head. His intense gaze studied every nuance of my facial expression while his hands caressed all my favorite places. Along with his throbbing penetration, his drawn features and still pose indicated that his body's need for release would soon overcome his restraint.

"Come with me, Coridan." I tightened my muscles around our one point of physical connection.

After a hoarse sound of surrender, Coridan stretched out full-length atop me. The weight of him shortened my breath. He nuzzled my ear, then whispered, "We belong together, Kalliope."

His sudden withdrawal and lunging thrust scattered my thoughts.

* * *

I awakened cuddled against Coridan's side. My splayed left hand covered the center of his muscularly defined chest. On my ring finger, the black opal surrounded by diamonds mesmerized me. I recognized the gemstones despite their being arranged in a new setting that was less elaborate than the one I had seen during Coridan's earlier marriage proposals.

Arctic air-conditioned atmosphere chilled my skin. Sometime during the pre-dawn hours, Coridan had shut the balcony doors in addition to placing this ring on my finger.

Coridan shifted from sleeping to wakefulness in an instant. He turned and pulled me flush against his body. We met face to face. Greeting me with a smile, he released me long enough to reach for the glass of water on the bedside table. He took a sip then offered one to me.

"Dr. Kalliope Cleary Ruskin," Coridan pronounced my name with solemn formality. "Will you and Cupcake grant Maya and me the honor of permanently and legally joining your lives with ours?" He framed my face between his palms. "Will you marry me, Kalliope Cleary Ruskin?"

He offered me everything I desired. I could choose him and keep myself.

"Yes."

WHO'S YOUR DADDY?

Dear Ezechiel,
By now I am a ghost, but I will
not haunt you. My treasure will
seek you. Please welcome him.
Forgive me and believe that no
malice was intended on my part.

Wilma Donald Mathias Witherspoon

Bryn, this is Lucian. By the time you return to modern civilization from the back of beyond, Mother will be interred at Elysian Plains. Wilma died in the hospital tonight. I know you will be upset with yourself for being inaccessible to me and Vernon, but don't. Just knowing that you will return to me soon consoles me.

Vernon Witherspoon, widower for seven days, watched his wife's son, Lucian Mathias, toss the first handful of earth atop the casket. Its rich mahogany finish gleamed obscenely in the bright spring sunshine,

127

which contributed nothing toward warming the senior gentleman's weary body and despondent heart. Only one more task to complete before all his promises were honored. After executing his own toss, Vernon stood beside Lucian to acknowledge the condolences from the parade of mourners.

Wilma Donald Mathias Witherspoon had managed to touch many lives during her fifty-year rise from housekeeper to society maven. The community had been as shocked as her husband and son when a minor cold became pneumonia, which ended her life after twelve days of valiant struggle.

Sometime during Vernon's musings, Lucian touched his arm.

"Here's the car, Vernon."

"What?" Vernon glanced from Lucian's long brown fingers wrapped around the black cashmere covering his forearm to the narrow graveled path where the limousine idled not far from Wilma's plot.

Lucian moved his hand up Vernon's arm and across his shoulder, securing the frail body within the shelter of his younger, larger, stronger frame. "Time for home."

He encouraged Vernon into action by taking a small step toward the open car door.

Vernon thought of the snug cottage he and Wilma had decorated ten years earlier when they decided to withdraw from the daily grind of the social whirl of their privileged set. The empty cottage was filled with the comforting possessions of a loving couple that no longer existed beyond photographs and a grieving man's fierce memories. He sighed and stepped toward the waiting car.

* * *

My darling, determined, stoic Lucian,

Every first look at you with your sage
eyes and man's body jars me for an
instant. You will always be my adored
baby boy.
Thank you for honoring my request that
you not contact your biological father
until after my death. Although life
generously offered me the love of
three good men, vanity and fear

prevented me from even the thought of confronting Ezechiel Burk's justifiable anger over my sins of omission regarding your existence.

I do not regret my choices— only the fact that you discovered the truth by browsing through a magazine. I should have told you sooner.

As you decide how to make peace with Ezechiel Burk, know that years ago he was

a man of integrity and wisdom even as a struggling young plumber. He will open his

heart to you if you offer him the same courtesy. I believe he would have loved and

cared for us if I had told him the truth of my pregnancy.

Thank you for being my beloved child,
Mama

"This is your handwriting, Vernon," he said to the still figure reclining on a chaise and bundled from neck to feet in a chenille throw. Lucian's de facto father of thirty-five years only nodded and smiled wanly in response.

Lucian waited and admonished himself not to panic about Vernon's increasing isolation from his physical environment. Yesterday's housecall by Vernon's physician had resulted in evidence of good vital statistics combined with alarming symptoms of extreme grief. Since Vernon refused to be hospitalized for observation, Lucian had arranged to reside with Vernon indefinitely.

Eyes mesmerized by the cheerful bounce of the flames in the stone fireplace, Vernon said, "The first time I proposed marriage, Wilma gave me sketchy details of your conception and Markus Mathias's eagerness to claim you as his own. 'Consider that, then ask me again,' she said." Vernon turned his head to meet Lucian's bland expression. "When I proposed marriage the following day, Wilma enthusiastically accepted. Having you in my life made me as happy as laying claim to Wilma. You're a fine boy, Lucian."

131

Lucian's mouth quirked into a brief lop-sided smile. At this point in his life he had been a man for more years than he had been a boy, but according to Vernon anyone under the age of fifty was a babe-in-arms. "Thank you, Vernon. You and Mama raised me well."

Markus Mathias, the man Lucian had believed to be his biological father until a year ago, had died of a stroke when Lucian was four years old. Mathias had been thirty-nine years older than his wife who became a wealthy widow. Lucian's mama met Vernon Witherspoon through negotiations to sell Mathias Antiquities to Witherspoon's Past Perfections. The sale stalled while the romance blossomed. After the wedding both concerns blended to become Mathias and Witherspoon Antiquities in order to preserve Lucian's nominal connection to the man listed as his father on his birth certificate.

As angry as Lucian had been upon discovering the truth of his biological father, he never forgot that his mother had chosen wisely with regard to the two men who had actively fathered him. Knowing vague details of her life of squalid poverty as the seventh child of ten made it easier for Lucian to speculate about his mama's motives for the choices she'd made.

"Vernon, if I seek to establish an active connection with Ezechiel Burk, will such action hurt you in any manner—no matter how slight?"

The concern shining from Lucian's eyes pricked Vernon's conscience. He needed to appear strong and capable in order for the dear boy to feel free to pursue his life. Vernon rearranged himself into an upright position against the bolster. "Lucian, pursue your life with my blessings. Anyone you accept into your heart will not hurt me. I've hoarded your affections for thirty-five years. Contact Ezechiel Burk. Go get your answers. You're always welcome wherever I am."

Lucian had no memory of ever hearing Vernon say, "I love you, son," but he had always known the statement to be true.

* * *

Bryn Kerry had experienced worse days, but she'd also experienced many better—much better—ones. The morning began without coffee, then advanced to two flat tires for which she saluted the genius of the inventor of canned tire inflator. The afternoon began with a mugging, but the thief stole only her best leather satchel (a style discontinued by the manufacturer) which contained her hemp-covered daily planner (personalized gift from one of her summer students at her sister's Math and Science Academy for Girls), fudge brownie lipstick (also discontinued, darnit!), and photocopies of a stack of preparatory studies reported to have been discovered beneath the floorboards of a 15, *rue de Peine* Paris studio once shared by Herman A. MacNeil and Henry Ossawa Tanner. Bryn rejoiced over the fact that her notebook PC, wireless phone, and wallet had been locked in the trunk of her car, and her keys in her pants pocket during the unpleasant event. The facsimiles of the sketches could easily be downloaded and reprinted.

At first glance the sketches appeared to be work drafts of Tanner's *The Battle of Life* and other canvases from his time at the *Academie Julien*: scenes of raucous artists among rows of easels; a large studio class obscured by smoke. There were a few pages of scenes from a fishing village. Rumors suggested that in preparing for Tanner's return to the U.S. after his collapse due to typhoid fever, his friends had been unable or had inadvertently failed to roll all of his canvases prior to his departure. Maybe MacNeil or someone else thought to preserve the canvases until Tanner's return. Bryn was jetlagged after days of a fact-finding wild goose chase in her efforts to unearth solid proof of the sketches' origins. Being late for an informal consultation with Ezechiel Burk about chunks of a sculpture found inside one of the units of an abandoned private storage building Burk Family Construction was renovating rounded out her day, and it was only 4:10 pm. She'd been in the U.S. for twelve hours and still hadn't managed to retrieve her messages.

Obeying the posted speed limits would get her from the police substation to the Burk job site in twenty-five minutes.

She arrived in seventeen.

* * *

Lucian Mathias's willingness to agree to a last-minute change of venue pleased Ezechiel although his curiosity about the man's reasons for using an intermediary to arrange a face-to-face meeting lessened somewhat compared to his interest in this new mystery discovered by his foreman.

Ezechiel resisted the urge to use his handkerchief to wipe the thick layer of dust from the dark face of the kneeling figure laid on its side. Electricity was dead and the space had been sealed for years prior to the start of renovations, so Ezechiel shone the beam of his battery operated portable spotlight over the fine details of face and form.

"Hello?"

Ezechiel heard the voice and wondered how his oldest child Alonzo had known to find him here. Did the boy's voice sound so throaty from the dust or allergies? "Straight back, then left, Son," he called as his arm arced to shine light at the door.

Lucian's steps faltered upon hearing the form of address. Had Ezechiel Burk discovered their connection and blithely accepted the existence of another offspring? Lucian doubted that scenario.

Lucian stepped into the open doorway and squinted into the bright light. "Mr. Ezechiel Burk?" he asked as he raised one hand to shield his eyes.

Ezechiel blinked his eyes and shook his head, but the image of his son Alonzo as he had looked prior to surviving the building collapse which had taken one eye and scarred one side of his face and most of his body did not waver. He concentrated his focus and noticed the differences: This man's muscle mass was leaner than Alonzo's. He was big without being bulky. Finally registering the man's averted gaze, Ezechiel directed the light toward the floor.

"Pardon me. Lucian Mathias?"

The indirect light concealed the color of his eyes, but the features of the man's face closely recreated Alonzo's former unblemished looks.

In an instant, the broad facts of the past fell into place in his mind. Now he understood Lucian's request to meet in person. "So you're Wilma's treasure. Welcome." He offered his free hand.

Shocked into continued silence, Lucian stepped forward to clasp the large, rough hand of the senior gentleman who smiled at him with watery eyes. Such easy acceptance seemed impossible to Lucian.

"Hello. Ezechiel? Are you aware that Mr. Vernon Witherspoon is napping in a car parked out front?" Her voice sounded closer with each word until she entered the storage unit. Her hot pink hardhat matched her tightly woven cable sweater over fitted tailored charcoal slacks. Her thick-soled boots left tracks to the right of those made by Lucian and Ezechiel. Her flashlight was small but powerful.

She directed her beam from one man's shoulder to the other. "Lucian?" she asked with equal parts joy and surprise. Their paths hadn't crossed personally or professionally in several months. Most often they met to cooperate, but occasionally they met in amicable competition in a race to acquire authentic works of art by African-American artists who were creating in the years of 1792 through 1950. Sometimes their clients placed bets on the outcome.

Ezechiel leaned forward to kiss Bryn's cheek, then Lucian gave her shoulders a one-armed squeeze, but he asked Ezechiel, "What have you found, Mr. Burk?" He squinted into the shadowy area behind the mirror image of himself in about twenty-five years.

"Call me Ezechiel, Lucian." It felt appropriate to delve into this mystery with his new son and the young woman who had become a daughter to him.

"Look," Ezechiel said to them before he caught the sculpture pieces in the beam of his spotlight.

Lucian and Bryn gasped softly.

Bryn spoke first. "Arrange for twenty-four hour discreet armed guard. Contact Jethro Glitnick at the Harlem Society for the Preservation of Original African-American Art. Tell Jeth what you think you have and he'll be on the next flight here. He lives and breathes Augusta Savage."

When she looked to Lucian for his reaction, Ezechiel said, "That's why I called you. I'll be the fool if this is some elaborate hoax."

Lucian said, "Bryn's right. Call Jethro. These fragments could be pieces of Savage's 1939 *Lift Every Voice and Sing*, which was smashed during the demolition after the New York World's Fair. You probably know she didn't have the funds to cast or store it."

139

Ezechiel nodded as the three of them stared at the figure of the kneeling young black man. Bryn aligned her beam with his. The stronger light allowed them to see three fingers of a large hand connected to the lower portion of a figure garbed in a robe.

Bryn's light shook from the excited tremor in her hand. Lucian gently wrapped his fingers around her delicate hand and guided her light into a slow sweep of the far wall and corner where they all saw a small wooden crate.

The low hum of Ezechiel's voice ended the silence. After completing three calls on his wireless, he said, "Armed security endorsed by the Guggenheim is en route. Glitnick will contact me whenever his flight arrives tonight. Lucian, is this Vernon Witherspoon with you?" Remembering Wilma's signature at the bottom of her note, he added, "Your stepfather?"

"He was married to Mama for thirty-five years."

"Your father then?"

"Yes."

Ezechiel decided to make peace with that answer later. "Would he appreciate the potential of this find?"

"Very much."

"Then go wake him. We have time."

* * *

"You and Vernon are," she poked his shoulder while she glared into his face, "staying with me for as long as you're in town. And your silent, tough guy pose doesn't intimidate me, Lucian Burk Mathias!"

From their position of standing a few feet away from the combatants, Vernon and Ezechiel watched with affection and amusement.

Hearing Lucian's full name jolted Ezechiel's heart, so he asked, "How long have they loved each other, Vernon?"

Vernon's chuckle became a cough when Lucian and Bryn glared his way. "Since Youth Orchestra in the third grade," he said softly without turning his head toward Ezechiel, knowing they'd both be severely reprimanded by their children if they burst into laughter. "Neither of them has been married nor come close to personal commitment with anyone else."

"What's their obstacle?"

"Bryn is the oldest of five girls. Her mother is currently with husband number five. Bryn feels obligated to set a strong example of how normal it is for a woman to be complete, fulfilled and at peace without clinging to a man. Lucian chooses to wait until the end of her self-imposed martyrdom to propose marriage, which should be soon. The last triplet graduates from medical school this December."

Ezechiel turned to meet Vernon's gaze. "Thank you for being a good father to Lucian."

Vernon smiled into the other man's eyes. "I simply followed Wilma's example with the boy. The day her attorney approached me about purchasing Mathias Antiquities enriched my life beyond my dreams."

* * *

Long and loud argument resulted in two unexpected, but much desired houseguests for Bryn, who tossed together a quick and tasty goulash for their late evening meal during which Lucian shared his story of an embarrassment of fathers. After Bryn chastised him for not confiding in her earlier, she gave the details of her possible Tanner sketches. Vernon, Lucian, and Bryn traded thoughts about the pieces of sculpture they had seen at the Burk work site. Although the possibility of having found significant portions of Savage's *The Harp* had sparked Vernon's interest like nothing else since his wife's death, he retired to bed immediately following a generous serving of homemade tart.

"He seems frail," Bryn said.

Since Bryn had yet to mention his mother's death, Lucian knew that she hadn't heard his message to her.

While she waited, Bryn's eyes noted the disturbing shadows in and around Lucian's fine dark eyes. She braced herself for an emotional hit.

"Mama died from complications resulting from pneumonia." On seeing the instantaneous tears and guilt in her eyes Lucian added, "There was no way to reach you before the service. I knew that before I called to leave the message."

Bryn hadn't thought to ask about Mrs. Witherspoon's whereabouts because the older woman always sent "her boys" on their treasure hunts as quality mega-testosterone time in which they enjoyed each other's company while she savored quiet time with herself. The tedious labors of establishing provenance had never appealed to Mrs. Witherspoon.

Bryn hopped from her seat and plopped into Lucian's lap without offering him the chance to reject her offer of physical comfort.

"Luc, how sad for you and Vernon. Tell me what happened." One hand rubbed circles across his back and the other caressed his jaw.

Lucian's watery eyes gazed into hers as if the sight of her supplied the strength to speak. "One day she had a persistent cough; the next day she was hospitalized. Two days after that she was comatose. She died a week later." His arms wrapped her tightly to his body. He pressed his face into the hollow of her neck and inhaled the fresh scent of her skin. "Maybe Mama would have fought harder to live if I'd never seen that magazine photo of Ezechiel Burk," he whispered.

"Maybe, Luc, but speculation will only add to your grief. Don't torture yourself with 'What if...?' Your mother loved you. Vernon loves you, and Ezechiel Burk seems anxious to know you, but willing to move at your pace."

Lucian's hands cinched her waist and his mouth covered her lips with ravenous intensity. Her unsteady perch forced Bryn to tighten her arms around his neck to prevent her body from tipping out of his lap under the force of his kisses.

When their lungs demanded more oxygen, Lucian asked, "Is this an invitation into your bed, Bryn?"

Her eyelids drifted up. She licked her lips as Lucian stared into her face. Years of being Lucian's lover had taught her that when under emotional duress he often preferred an initial hard and fast penetration before settling into more leisurely love making. Bryn said, "You're invited into my body. The bed is optional."

Lucian shoved back his chair, dumped Bryn onto her back on the smooth walnut surface of her antique dining table, and loomed above her. His strong fingers seized her hips dragging them to the edge of the table. His wide stance spread her legs until her thighs trembled with strain.

"It's been a long three months, Bryn."

The harshness of his voice would have threatened her if she hadn't known him for most of her life.

"I know, Luc."

Lucian slapped his left hand near her right shoulder, then his right hand near her left shoulder. Slowly, he lowered his chest until the weight of his upper body flattened her breasts.

"Hurry, Bryn."

Lucian's kisses interfered with her ability to concentrate on unfastening his pants then hers after he narrowed his stance, but she managed. Lucian groaned in relief at the release of the pressure on his erection. Their lips disconnected when she wiggled her hips to push down her pants. Her agile fingers gently clasped his penis and guided it toward her very wet center. As soon as the engorged cap touched her damp folds Lucian's hips surged forward until he was deeply seated within the tight fit of her body. Bryn's hips teetered at the table edge and her legs dangled, unable to curl around his hips due to the restraint of her trousers pushed halfway down her thighs. Her back arched off the table and she breathed deeply through her mouth in an attempt to accept his presence without pain.

Lucian's weight lifted from her chest when he reached down to remove her pants. One at a time, Lucian picked up Bryn's legs and placed them over his forearms. She lay there completely exposed and vulnerable to his powerful body. He watched her eyes, waiting for their expression to shift from cautious acceptance to passionate desire. Gradually the color of her eyes deepened while her breathing shifted from frantic panting to deep sighing. Her vaginal muscles no longer worked to expel him; they clutched to keep him.

Lucian bent forward at the waist folding her legs between their bodies.

"Lift your sweater, Bryn," he said twice before she gathered the resources to act.

Lucian's ferocious smile revealed his pleasure in seeing her round breasts swathed in hot pink lace. He teased her and himself with small forward and back shifts of his hips. Bryn's fingers snagged his shirt pulling him closer.

She glared at him. "Lucian!"

His wider smile reflected a moment of humor. Bryn Kerry had been bossing him since their first encounter in the strings section of Youth Orchestra.

He settled into a hard, steady rhythm of thrust and withdrawal.

147

* * *

"You can forgive her so easily, Ezechiel?" Odessa met her husband's gaze reflected in the mirror above her vanity table.

He continued smoothing cocoa butter cream into her shoulders and across her back. "Wilma Donald loved me. I was her first lover. At the time I barely generated enough profit to shelter, clothe, and feed myself, much less a wife and babe. Looking back, I remember how hard she worked to bring the struggling company that I had inherited from my father to the attention of potential clients she met through being Mathias's housekeeper. Then I resented her interference, but now I realize that she knew or suspected that she was pregnant." Ezechiel straightened the sleeves of her nightdress.

His wife spun on the tufted stool. They were eye-to-eye because Ezechiel knelt. Odessa held his face between her capable hands. "Invite him to the melee we call Sunday dinner. I'll call the children to prepare them for his resemblance to the way Alonzo used to look."

Odessa looked into her husband's eyes and recognized his pain while she thanked Wilma Donald's spirit for the choices she made that had allowed her and her children with Ezechiel to be the primary focus of his life.

"You're not hurt by this or disappointed in me, O.?"

"No." She leaned forward to press a friendly kiss to his mouth. "According to what you've said, Lucian Mathias's mother had been married for a year by the time you and I were introduced. Your past with her doesn't harm or shame me in any way."

Ezechiel's eyes glistened above his brilliant smile. He rose and claimed his wife's hand leading her to their bed.

* * *

Lucian and Bryn stood on the wraparound porch of the elder Burks' suburban home.

"Thank you for coming with me, Bryn."

"Thanks for inviting me."

He turned toward her. "You're not here as penance for being unavailable during Mama's funeral are you?"

149

Bryn juggled the gift basket of preserves and beeswax candles into the crook of her arm, then clasped his hand and squeezed. "Being with you is never penance, Luc. Ring the bell."

A cherubic little brown face appeared in a window to the left of the door. She waved until fingers wrapped around her shoulders and pulled her away leaving a swish of drapery in her wake.

Lucian rang the bell.

* * *

Introductions, drinks, and appetizers went more smoothly than any of the adults had imagined.

"Where's Vernon?" Ezechiel asked once they had settled into their places at the huge round dining table.

"He and an old classmate are reminiscing at Bryn's house while inhaling her pot of crab bisque soup," Lucian said.

Ezechiel turned to Bryn. "As many times as you and I have met to confer about objects found at my job sites and you never noticed how much I resemble your boyfriend whose middle name is Burk, Ms. Bryn Kerry, observer of all minutiae?"

Bryn's sheepish grin charmed them all. "To me, Lucian's looks are unique. Before today I'd never met or seen any of your children. You and I always meet at construction sites." She looked across the table at the striking man with the eye patch and facial scars who steadily returned her gaze. "Obviously, seeing you, Alonzo, would have inspired questions about Lucian's ancestry."

* * *

Lucian watched his new siblings and their mates interact with each other and with Ezechiel and Odessa Burk. Although they'd had two weeks to reconcile themselves to his existence, he still marveled at the sincerity of their welcome. Last month he'd been an only child. Today he had four siblings, sisters-in-law, a de facto brother-in-law, a niece, and two people willing to love him as their child.

"Uncle Luc?"

Lucian inclined his head toward the little girl who had shadowed him since he stepped inside the house. "Yes, Maya?"

"I'm very happy Granddaddy found you. Will you please be my show and tell this week?" she whispered.

Coridan laughed. "It's official, Lucian. My daughter has already taken Alonzo, Georgette, and Mordecai. Every week five students are encouraged to invite a guest to explain the details of his or her career. They're only ten students in her class, so every other week Maya presses someone into service. We'll understand if prior obligations prevent you from participating." He directed a stern look at his daughter. "Won't we, Maya?"

"Yes, Daddy," she said because his look meant that her agreement was very important.

Lucian said, "Vernon and I will be in town indefinitely. If you," he raised his eyes toward Ezechiel, "and Jethro don't mind, Vernon would enjoy helping you establish provenance for your most recent find. And yes," he said to his patient young niece, "I would enjoy being your show and tell, Maya. Thank you for asking."

Coridan said, "We'll fax the guidelines to you at Bryn's." He looked to Bryn for confirmation of his assumptions.

* * *

After dessert, the Burk men, R.J., and Lucian filled Odessa's spacious kitchen. Ezechiel loaded the dishwasher with pots and pans. Mordecai washed the china, silver, and crystal while R.J. dried. Coridan returned each item to its assigned location.

"Five. Four. Three," Mordecai said.

"What?" Lucian whispered, glancing around for signs of unusual activity in the kitchen designed from a gourmet chef's dream.

Mordecai's smile broadened although he shook his head at Lucian. "Two. One."

Bearing a crystal water goblet in one hand, Odessa Burk strolled into the room. "Here, boys, I'm finished." Her keen gaze noted each man's position and which of her valuable possessions he held and how he held it. A soft smile shaped her lips when she placed the goblet in the sudsy water in the center section of her triple cook sink.

"Come join us in the hot spot when you've finished." Her regal bearing carried her from their presence with admirable grace.

Lucian smiled and waited for details while the other men laughed aloud.

"Twenty-five years of this tradition and she still doesn't trust us completely," Alonzo said.

"Hey, twenty-four years ago Coridan dropped Grandma Nelson's serving platter," Mordecai said.

"Accidentally, baby brother," Coridan growled in response to his sibling's taunt.

Ezechiel started the wash cycle, then turned toward Lucian. "Next time you come you'll be assigned kitchen duty, too. O. doesn't completely trust us, but she endorses equitable division of labor. If you don't cook, you clean.

"O.'s invitation to join them means that the serious woman talk is finished. The hot spot is the family room with the eight by eight stone fireplace. Georgette named it during our first winter here. Questions?"

Lucian shook his head.

* * *

Lucian sat amid the luxurious sofa cushions covered in heathered flannel. Maya lay sleeping draped across his legs. Stephanie Jeffers eased into place beside him.

"Pardon Maya's presumptuous actions; experience has taught her that we all live to provide her with comfort. Since you're her new uncle she has to give you a test run as her personal cushion." Stephanie glanced down at the sleeping child who sighed and drooled on Lucian's tailored trousers. She addressed Lucian's shell-shocked expression with a sympathetic smile. "Being accepted by the Burks is overwhelming, but very real and enduring, Lucian." She covered his hand where it rested gently against Maya's chaotic mass of hair. "They will encourage you to set the pace for being incorporated into their lives." She gave a quick squeeze before she rose from her seat. Her attention swerved across the room. "Now I'm off to rescue your beloved from the tender inquisition of Jessamine and Kalliope who never follow Georgette's example of discretion. They're probably pumping Bryn for information I wouldn't let them get earlier. Send the drycleaning bill to Coridan. He always reimburses for wear and tear on Maya's human cushions," she said as she headed across the room.

"Sometimes he pays in trade," Mordecai said without taking his eyes from the chessboard. "Find out if Bryn needs any plumbing maintenance. CEO Burk will dispatch a crew."

Coridan didn't bother to comment since years of being teased by his brothers had inured him to their lack of deference regarding his position at the top of the Burk Family Enterprises hierarchy.

"We've invited Bryn to lunch with us next month," Kalliope said to forestall Stephanie's scolding when she reached their tight circle.

"So stop with that disapproving librarian's scowl," Jessamine said. "Georgette has derailed all our attempts to interrogate Bryn about her relationship with Lucian."

All the women looked directly at Bryn's platinum ring decorated with Latin script. Lucian wore a masculine version of the same design.

"Good," Stephanie said to her sisters-in-law, then said to Bryn, "Lucian's exhibiting signs of sensory overload. Take him home. Give him a nightcap and put him to bed. Tell him to call Mama O. when he's ready for round two."

Bryn started a round of farewell hugs and kisses among the women. From the corner of her eye, she saw Alonzo approach Lucian. She stepped in the opposite direction, toward Ezechiel.

* * *

"Before the accident, you and I could have passed as identical twins," Alonzo said after he sat beside Lucian and exchanged a thick photo album for the precious burden of Maya's weight. Maya snuggled into the bulkier embrace without waking. The stuffed book fell open across Lucian's thighs. He ignored its allure.

Alonzo sat still while Lucian's perfect eyes in his perfect face examined the distorted reflection of Alonzo's scarred visage. His black eye patch covered the eyelid sown over the sunken empty socket.

Lucian noted the similarities and differences between this familiar stranger's face and his own. "Does seeing me hurt you, Alonzo?"

Alonzo's monocular gaze swept the room full of loved ones who did a poor job of pretending not to listen. "You have courage to ask the question they want answered."

Lucian slid forward and angled his body toward Alonzo, who smiled into his new brother's face. Thinking of himself as the oldest of five would require some adjustment.

"If the sight of me causes you pain, I am willing to know Ezechiel separately from the extended Burk family. I have no desire to infringe on your prior claim to the Burks. Vernon has been a good father to me. He and Mama provided me with love and a solid family. Do you understand what I'm saying, Alonzo?"

Alonzo immediately understood that he would benefit from being kin to this generous man.

Generosity deserved to be met with honesty. "My first glimpse of you was disconcerting even though Dad had done his best to prepare me. But now, after hours of looking at you I feel glad that, beyond old photographs, my face still exists as it was before the accident. So thank you for your consideration, and believe that all of us anticipate being in your company as often as you will allow."

They drifted into discussion of easier topics before Lucian followed Bryn's example and started his own round of farewells.

* * *

Entering Bryn's quiet home lit only by the night safety lights, Lucian called, "Vernon?" as he followed Bryn toward the hall table where a note lay propped against her brass key basket.

By peering over her shoulder, Lucian read that Vernon had accepted Stanley's invitation to spend several days with him. When Bryn turned to offer comment, Lucian framed her face between his hands and kissed her until she sank into the strength of his body. His eyes remained open. He did nothing to hide his physical and emotional need for her attention.

"Bryn," he whispered her name between kisses to her closed eyes, nose, prominent cheeks, and round chin.

She heard the confusion and entreaty underscoring the tenor of his voice. She claimed his hand and led him to her bedroom.

* * *

Knowing that Lucian felt as if his family life was beyond his control, Bryn surrendered herself to Lucian's desires. Nearly thirty years of being his nemesis, friend, and finally, lover had taught her to trust him.

She did not panic when he silently loosened his clothes while she stood where he had left her beside the bed. Her curiosity piqued when he moved her antique cheval mirror to face the foot of her bed before he came to her and unceremoniously stripped her bare.

Lucian's eyes devoured her abundant physical beauty. He waited for her to question him, but she only smiled and opened her arms to him. Her comparable height allowed her to gaze directly into his eyes.

"I love you, Lucian. By whatever name you are called; no matter who offers you claim to their family, I love you."

Bryn loosened her arms from him and collapsed across her bed on her back with her arms flung above her head. "Come to bed, Lucian."

Relief made him laugh aloud. No matter the situation, he could always rely on Bryn to boss him.

* * *

"Lucian," Bryn gasped softly against his thumb laid across the width of her tongue.

The mirror's reflection of their position at the foot of the bed showed Lucian's finger disappearing within the glistening folds of her sex. With her legs draped over his knees, she had a clear view of her neatly groomed mons and labia. She watched Lucian as he watched her hands fondle her breasts and tug at her distended nipples. The slumberous look in his eyes contradicted the insistent prod of his erection against the small of her back. His hand at her mouth drifted over her face and neck in a brief caress as it lowered to the sensitive and vulnerable spot between her legs. The fingers of one hand spread her folds while another finger of the other hand gently eased inside her for shallow penetration. Her clitoris received no attention.

Lucian clamped his thighs tightly about Bryn's hips to prevent her from thrusting. Panting heavily, she arched her spine into a deep curve and wiggled around the tight fit of his fingers. He recognized the signs of her imminent orgasm.

In rapid succession Lucian withdrew his fingers, dumped her from his lap, and tossed her onto her back leaving her gasping up at him and trembling at the edge of orgasm. Lucian dragged his weight over her body. After clasping one of her hands in each of his, Lucian gathered her hands into one of his and used the other to place the head of his penis at the gate to her womb. Slowly, he pushed forward. Even as aroused as Bryn was, her body worked to accept him. Seconds later she squirmed around the fullness of his presence. Soft sounds of minor discomfort escaped her parted lips. Lucian held himself very still and watched her watery eyes for the truth.

"Too much, Bryn?"

He waited.

"Open your legs a bit," she said quietly.

He realized that her legs were trapped between his, increasing her difficulty in accepting him. Bryn smiled when he spread his legs until they no longer sandwiched hers. The adjustment pushed him deeper. Bryn's pelvis rose to meet his. Lucian withdrew, then returned with controlled power. He hooked his hands under her shoulders to provide more leverage. He settled atop her and looked into her eyes. They both groaned.

"If we ever conceive, Bryn," he said after several deep breaths. "Promise to tell me—regardless of the state of our relationship. Promise me, Bryn." His voice wavered in pitch and volume. She felt the fine trembling of his tautly held body as if her own limbs were shaking.

Bryn knew that the reality of her fertile years being history would not console Luc. She wrapped her arms around his sleek shoulders developed from years of swimming laps. His utter despair prompted her to say, "I promise you, Lucian." She smiled into his pensive stare. "Your mother left Ezechiel Burk because she feared he wouldn't be able to provide for her and her child." A small shift of his weight forced her to suck in a deep breath. "I know that you can and would willingly provide for me and a child in addition to my ability to provide for myself. Judgment of unwed mothers has changed since your mother's pregnancy. There would be no reason for me to withhold the truth from you, Lucian. I would be happy to share such news with you."

Some of the tension evident in Lucian's face eased. He kissed her, his tongue sweeping the warm sweet interior of her mouth with the purpose of staking irrevocable claim.

* * *

Sitting in Lucian's lap while they lingered over the three courses of breakfast Lucian had prepared, Bryn cupped his cheek in her palm and turned his face to hers. Shadows of strain and confusion had faded from his eyes although tension still thrummed the limbs that cradled her close to his chest.

"Multiple sources suggest that Henry Ossawa Tanner contributed murals to a mosque that was being rebuilt during the time of his travels in Cairo in 1897. The mosque had been looted and vandalized. Today it's not used, but there are curious parties in Egypt and the U.S. who want the rumors thoroughly investigated...."

Lucian heard her words, but focused on the visual appeal of her lips. Memories of the manner in which her mouth had moved over his body during the night generated instant physical response.

Bryn leaned forward to rub her nose against his.

"Stop fantasizing about my mouth, Lucian. Pay attention."

His tongue licked out at the drop of boysenberry preserves smeared at the corner of her mouth before his gaze traveled over the sweeping curves of her cheeks and nose to collide with the merry twinkling of her eyes. He smiled as he waited.

"I just invited you to leave with me for Cairo in three weeks. Vernon, too, if he cares to join us."

Lucian considered his immediate desire to accept against Vernon's emotional and physical frailty. He knew that Vernon would correctly interpret Lucian's refusal to go without him as a show of concern for the older man's health. Vernon would be annoyed. His disposition would shift from mildly irritable to cantankerous in an instant.

Bryn resisted her desire to prod Lucian into answering. He had always been a meticulous planner.

She easily read the progression of his thoughts as they flickered behind his eyes.

She wasn't surprised when he said, "Being with you in Cairo, Bryn, is a combination too potent to resist. Whether Vernon accompanies us or doesn't, I'll need to make arrangements for him." Lucian groaned at the thought of making plans for a man who would resist all his efforts before granting his cooperation. "Hale can be trusted to continue his supervision of Mathias and Witherspoon's daily operations. My passport is current."

For the next hour they discussed details of the excursion.

* * *

Turning at the sound of Odessa's entrance, Ezechiel said, "Bon voyage, Bryn," and disconnected.

Odessa balanced her weight on the arm of the extra-large wingchair that supported her husband's slouching figure.

"They leave in two days. Vernon is already settled into his friend's guest cottage." Ezechiel's deep sigh echoed his sadness due to the fact that he had not seen or spoken to Lucian since the family dinner weeks earlier. Honoring Lucian's desires as his first priority in their tenuous relationship opposed his need to badger his new son into maintaining more frequent contact. Ezechiel's hand idly clasped his wife's warm round thigh.

"Ezechiel, in the past two months Lucian has buried his mother, met his biological father for the first time, and gone from being an only child to the oldest of five in addition to being on the fringes of an historic art find."

Jethro Glitnick and his team hovered on the brink of providing irrefutable evidence that the sculpture pieces found at the Burk Family Construction site were from Augusta Savage's *Lift Every Voice and Sing*.

"Add Lucian's concerns about Vernon's health to the mix, and the boy must be feeling emotionally punch drunk." Odessa found it impossible to close her heart to someone whose appearance so closely resembled that of her beloved unruly children. She covered her husband's hand, then smiled into his morose expression. "Eventually, your patience will be rewarded."

* * *

"Thank you for making time to see me before your departure tomorrow, Lucian."

Neither man bothered pursuing more small talk. Ezechiel's eyes drank in every feature of the familiar stranger's appearance as he poured opaque black coffee into two china mugs.

Lucian kept his dark gaze averted when he said, "Bryn asked me what purpose avoiding you was serving. She also said she didn't want my regrets to ruin our time in Cairo." One side of his mouth kicked up. He gazed into a wiser set of his own eyes. "Bryn knows me very well."

Many questions occurred to Ezechiel, but he remained silently encouraging. Each man raised his mug to his mouth.

"I'm so angry at Mama and you for choices you made that cannot be changed. But I also feel like an ingrate because Mama chose honorable and loving men three times in her life, and I always benefited. Meeting you and seeing you interact with your family have convinced me that you would have loved me if you had known about me." Lucian abandoned his mug to a small marble accent table. His hands shook when he raised them to rake his fingers across his scalp. "Still, waves of anger roil through me until I feel nauseated," he whispered.

Ezechiel internally debated his response until he decided that one word from him would spring Lucian's desperately necessary emotional release. "Son, I— "

Lucian's hands dropped from his face and his eyes rose from the contemplation of his knees. "Son?" he asked in a rigidly controlled voice. "Until last year only two people had legitimate right to claim that connection to me: a man who died before I could acquire solid memories of him, and Mama. Then those photographs of you and all the Burks in *Emerge* made sense of my middle name and physical attributes." He sneered into Ezechiel's open expression. "When I was a boy I would have granted Vernon the right to call me son, but he always told me he didn't want to displace my affection for my real father. To me he's always been my real father."

Ezechiel recognized a boy's teary heartbreak trapped within the man's dry-eyed angst. He wondered how much revelation about Wilma's family history would console Lucian. He speculated that his mother had revealed very few details to her only child.

"As the seventh child of ten, Wilma Donald was never the original owner of any material item provided by her parents." Ezechiel remembered the care with which she had handled the inexpensive trinkets and garments he had given her as gifts during their courtship. "By the time she and her younger siblings were school age, Wilma believed that her parents viewed them only as burdens that drained the family's meager resources. She would not have wanted that life for you, Lucian. I think she wanted priority claim to your love. I think marrying Markus Mathias gave her everything she needed at that time." No need to add that Mathias's childless ex-wives had whispered of sterility. Whispers that the community gossips had attributed to resentment. "They moved soon after the wedding."

"Who left whom, Ezechiel, you or Mama?"

He chose not to reciprocate the belligerent tone. "One night Wilma came to the boarding house to tell me she was ready to settle down. Her employer had proposed. I thanked her for telling me personally and wished her well. We waited silently at the bus stop until her bus came. Two weeks later I read the wedding announcement."

"What if— "

Ezechiel spread his hands and shrugged. "What if I had questioned her motives for the visit? For the sudden marriage? What if I had recognized the clues she'd been giving me for weeks? Those questions and thousands more have haunted me since you and I first met, Lucian. I do know that I'm grateful to Wilma and her husbands for loving and caring for you. You're a fine man. Everything else will require time to sort." Ezechiel waited, hoping his revelations had struck perfect balance between consoling his son and protecting the man's memories of his mother.

With a deep breath, Lucian's belligerence fled, leaving only exhaustion. "Bryn and anger are my only constants. Everything else has a surreal quality that unnerves me." He stared into the older man's eyes, willing to accept any help he was willing to offer.

171

"Rely on Bryn's love for you. Go to Cairo with an open heart. Search for treasure. Ride your anger to its source and disarm it. Vernon, Odessa, the children, and I will be here when you return, Lucian." There were so many more words he wanted to say, but Ezechiel rose from his seat when he saw Lucian's eyelids drift shut. He stepped close enough to brush his palm over the shorn waves of Lucian's hair.

* * *

Ezechiel detoured to Bryn's home office en route to the exit.

"How long will you keep Lucian occupied in Cairo, Bryn?" he asked quietly from his stance near the doorjamb.

She turned from her final inventory of relevant reference books. Her smile acknowledged the truth of his implied meaning. "A month, maybe more if that's what it takes for Lucian to sleep for more than two hours in a stretch." Her tone challenged him to ridicule her goal.

"He's sleeping right now. Nodded off in that monstrosity of a chair in your library."

Bryn leaned forward. "It was a gift from a client who was enormously pleased not to be fleeced in a swindle centered on an Edmonia Lewis work. She's a close friend to my mother, so it seemed unwise to refuse it."

Ezechiel smiled sadly when Bryn winked at him. He responded to her earlier statement. "Keep Lucian away for as long as it takes for him to be at peace with this situation. Odessa and I will stay in touch with Vernon; pester him to manage his health." He watched his fingers manipulate the buttons of his overcoat. "We would enjoy receiving postcards as frequently as you and Lucian could manage. He looked up to find Bryn standing very close to him.

She hugged his stiff body tightly, then pulled back to gaze into his face. "Lucian already loves you and the Burks; already wants you in his life, but he's confused and afraid. He's still mourning his mama and feeling betrayed by her and Vernon, too. The scents, sounds, textures, and legacy of Cairo should help him put his life in perspective. We might retrace Tanner's tour of northern Africa. Lucian and I have always been a capable team, Ezechiel."

He pressed his dry lips against Bryn's warm brown cheek. "Happy hunting and travel safely," he said. "Thank you for encouraging this opportunity for us to speak before your departure. Your love for him is fierce and true, Bryn."

Ezechiel released her and retreated down the hall. Seconds later her security system indicated the opening and closing of the front door.

About the Author

Cardyn Brooks is a bibliophile with a Bachelor of Arts degree in English. Her constant search for engaging erotic fiction that features non-stereotypical characters with voracious sensual appetites inspired her to write stories she desired to read—stories about adults as powerful sexual beings who pursue their sensual needs while juggling the demands of home, work, family, and friends.

She lives on the east coast of the United States with her family.

www.ingramcontent.com/pod-product-compliance
Lightning Source LLC
Chambersburg PA
CBHW020417290526
45785CB00002B/601